Jiffy Journal

Healthy Emotional Lifestyle

www.jiffyjournal.com

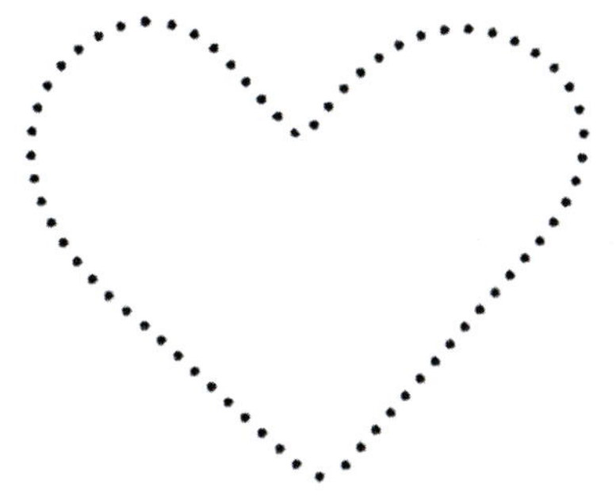

Emotional well-being, intelligence and growth contribute to all aspects of life. Jiffy Journal® is a quick, easy way to acknowledge feelings, guide behavior and build a history of valuable information.

Circle the day of the week, fill in the month, year and time. And you have begun building a valuable history. Check off what applies to you, while guided to write further thoughts, feelings and actions. Knowing how you feel helps to make happy, healthy decisions.

Jiffy Journal®, The journal worth keeping

☐ Sunny ☐ partly cloudy ☒ cloudy ☐ rain ☐ Snow

-10 zero 10's 20's 30's 40's 50's 60's 70's 80's 90's 100's
☐   ☐   ☐   ☐   ☒   ☐   ☐   ☐   ☐   ☐   ☐   ☐

I FEEL

- Happy
- Confident
- Excited
- Enthusiastic
- Powerful
- Fantastic
- Lucky
- Hopeful
- Content
- Focused
- Good
- Grateful
- Confused
- Sad
- Ashamed
- Lonely
- Frustrated
- Angry
- Hurt
- Jealous
- Exhausted
- Overwhelmed
- Tired
- Scared
- Feminine

I Spent most of today with
School & I was kinda mad at everyone but not at the same time like idk & then I got to see bae jana lol.

What I like the most today
Seeing Jana & the fact I get to skip hmrw to study & take a mental health day which I rly need.

What I like the least today
Feeling jealous & feeling like ppl don't like me but they do at the same time just not enough to be in the "__" like idk it's confusing.

TODAY'S CHOICES

Physically	Mentally	Spiritually
☐ working	☐ reading	☐ meditating
☐ exercising	☐ doing a project	☐ praying
☐ shopping	☐ practicing	☐ with nature
☐ gardening	☐ organizing	☐ being challenged
☐ traveling	☐ thinking	☐ with family + friends
☐ playing	☐ planning	☐ relaxing

More thoughts...etc.....

SMTWTFS _________________________ 20___ ___ AM PM

☐ Sunny ☐ partly cloudy ☐ cloudy ☐ rain ☐ Snow

-10 zero 10's 20's 30's 40's 50's 60's 70's 80's 90's 100's
☐   ☐   ☐   ☐   ☐   ☐   ☐   ☐   ☐   ☐   ☐   ☐

I FEEL

Happy
Confident
Excited
Enthusiastic
Powerful
Fantastic
Lucky
Hopeful
Content
Focused
Good
Grateful
Confused
Sad
Ashamed
Lonely
Frustrated
Angry
Hurt
Jealous
Exhausted
Overwhelmed
Tired
Scared

I Spent most of today with

____
____
____
____
____

What I like the most today

____
____
____
____

What I like the least today

____
____
____

TODAY'S CHOICES

Physically	Mentally	Spiritually
☐ working	☐ reading	☐ meditating
☐ exercising	☐ doing a project	☐ praying
☐ shopping	☐ practicing	☐ with nature
☐ gardening	☐ organizing	☐ being challenged
☐ traveling	☐ thinking	☐ with family + friends
☐ playing	☐ planning	☐ relaxing

More thoughts...etc.....

SMTWTFS _________________ 20 __ __ AM PM

☐ Sunny   ☐ partly cloudy   ☐ cloudy   ☐ rain   ☐ Snow

-10 zero 10's 20's 30's 40's 50's 60's 70's 80's 90's 100's
☐   ☐   ☐   ☐   ☐   ☐   ☐   ☐   ☐   ☐   ☐   ☐

I FEEL
Happy
Confident
Excited
Enthusiastic
Powerful
Fantastic
Lucky
Hopeful
Content
Focused
Good
Grateful
Confused
Sad
Ashamed
Lonely
Frustrated
Angry
Hurt
Jealous
Exhausted
Overwhelmed
Tired
Scared

I Spent most of today with

____
____
____
____
____

What I like the most today

____
____
____
____

What I like the least today

____
____
____

TODAY'S CHOICES

Physically	Mentally	Spiritually
☐ working	☐ reading	☐ meditating
☐ exercising	☐ doing a project	☐ praying
☐ shopping	☐ practicing	☐ with nature
☐ gardening	☐ organizing	☐ being challenged
☐ traveling	☐ thinking	☐ with family + friends
☐ playing	☐ planning	☐ relaxing

More thoughts...etc.....

SMTWTFS _____________ 20___ ___ AM / PM

☐ Sunny ☐ partly cloudy ☐ cloudy ☐ rain ☐ Snow

-10	zero	10's	20's	30's	40's	50's	60's	70's	80's	90's	100's
☐	☐	☐	☐	☐	☐	☐	☐	☐	☐	☐	☐

I FEEL

- Happy
- Confident
- Excited
- Enthusiastic
- Powerful
- Fantastic
- Lucky
- Hopeful
- Content
- Focused
- Good
- Grateful
- Confused
- Sad
- Ashamed
- Lonely
- Frustrated
- Angry
- Hurt
- Jealous
- Exhausted
- Overwhelmed
- Tired
- Scared

I Spent most of today with

____

____

____

____

____

What I like the most today

____

____

____

____

What I like the least today

____

____

____

TODAY'S CHOICES

Physically	Mentally	Spiritually
☐ working	☐ reading	☐ meditating
☐ exercising	☐ doing a project	☐ praying
☐ shopping	☐ practicing	☐ with nature
☐ gardening	☐ organizing	☐ being challenged
☐ traveling	☐ thinking	☐ with family + friends
☐ playing	☐ planning	☐ relaxing

More thoughts...etc.....

SMTWTFS ________________ 20___ ___ AM PM

☐ Sunny ☐ partly cloudy ☐ cloudy ☐ rain ☐ Snow

-10 zero 10's 20's 30's 40's 50's 60's 70's 80's 90's 100's
☐   ☐   ☐   ☐   ☐   ☐   ☐   ☐   ☐   ☐   ☐   ☐

I FEEL
Happy
Confident
Excited
Enthusiastic
Powerful
Fantastic
Lucky
Hopeful
Content
Focused
Good
Grateful
Confused
Sad
Ashamed
Lonely
Frustrated
Angry
Hurt
Jealous
Exhausted
Overwhelmed
Tired
Scared

I Spent most of today with

____
____
____
____
____

What I like the most today

____
____
____
____

What I like the least today

____
____
____
____

TODAY'S CHOICES

Physically	Mentally	Spiritually
☐ working	☐ reading	☐ meditating
☐ exercising	☐ doing a project	☐ praying
☐ shopping	☐ practicing	☐ with nature
☐ gardening	☐ organizing	☐ being challenged
☐ traveling	☐ thinking	☐ with family + friends
☐ playing	☐ planning	☐ relaxing

More thoughts...etc.....

SMTWTFS _________________ 20___ ___ AM PM

☐ Sunny   ☐ partly cloudy   ☐ cloudy   ☐ rain   ☐ Snow

-10 zero 10's 20's 30's 40's 50's 60's 70's 80's 90's 100's
☐   ☐   ☐   ☐   ☐   ☐   ☐   ☐   ☐   ☐   ☐   ☐

I FEEL

Happy
Confident
Excited
Enthusiastic
Powerful
Fantastic
Lucky
Hopeful
Content
Focused
Good
Grateful
Confused
Sad
Ashamed
Lonely
Frustrated
Angry
Hurt
Jealous
Exhausted
Overwhelmed
Tired
Scared

I Spent most of today with

____
____
____
____
____

What I like the most today

____
____
____
____

What I like the least today

____
____
____

TODAY'S CHOICES

Physically	Mentally	Spiritually
☐ working	☐ reading	☐ meditating
☐ exercising	☐ doing a project	☐ praying
☐ shopping	☐ practicing	☐ with nature
☐ gardening	☐ organizing	☐ being challenged
☐ traveling	☐ thinking	☐ with family + friends
☐ playing	☐ planning	☐ relaxing

More thoughts...etc.....

SMTWTFS _________________ 20___ ___

AM
PM

☐ Sunny   ☐ partly cloudy   ☐ cloudy   ☐ rain   ☐ Snow

-10 zero 10's 20's 30's 40's 50's 60's 70's 80's 90's 100's
☐   ☐   ☐   ☐   ☐   ☐   ☐   ☐   ☐   ☐   ☐   ☐

I FEEL

Happy
Confident
Excited
Enthusiastic
Powerful
Fantastic
Lucky
Hopeful
Content
Focused
Good
Grateful
Confused
Sad
Ashamed
Lonely
Frustrated
Angry
Hurt
Jealous
Exhausted
Overwhelmed
Tired
Scared

I Spent most of today with

____
____
____
____

What I like the most today

____
____
____
____

What I like the least today

____
____
____
____

TODAY'S CHOICES

Physically	Mentally	Spiritually
☐ working	☐ reading	☐ meditating
☐ exercising	☐ doing a project	☐ praying
☐ shopping	☐ practicing	☐ with nature
☐ gardening	☐ organizing	☐ being challenged
☐ traveling	☐ thinking	☐ with family + friends
☐ playing	☐ planning	☐ relaxing

More thoughts...etc.....

SMTWTFS _____________________ 20___ ___ AM PM

☐ Sunny ☐ partly cloudy ☐ cloudy ☐ rain ☐ Snow

-10 zero 10's 20's 30's 40's 50's 60's 70's 80's 90's 100's
☐   ☐   ☐   ☐   ☐   ☐   ☐   ☐   ☐   ☐   ☐   ☐

I FEEL
Happy
Confident
Excited
Enthusiastic
Powerful
Fantastic
Lucky
Hopeful
Content
Focused
Good
Grateful
Confused
Sad
Ashamed
Lonely
Frustrated
Angry
Hurt
Jealous
Exhausted
Overwhelmed
Tired
Scared

I Spent most of today with
____
____
____
____
____

What I like the most today
____
____
____
____

What I like the least today
____
____
____
____

TODAY'S CHOICES

Physically	Mentally	Spiritually
☐ working	☐ reading	☐ meditating
☐ exercising	☐ doing a project	☐ praying
☐ shopping	☐ practicing	☐ with nature
☐ gardening	☐ organizing	☐ being challenged
☐ traveling	☐ thinking	☐ with family + friends
☐ playing	☐ planning	☐ relaxing

More thoughts...etc.....

SMTWTFS _______________ 20___ ___

AM
PM

☐ Sunny ☐ partly cloudy ☐ cloudy ☐ rain ☐ Snow

-10 zero 10's 20's 30's 40's 50's 60's 70's 80's 90's 100's
☐ ☐ ☐ ☐ ☐ ☐ ☐ ☐ ☐ ☐ ☐ ☐

I FEEL
Happy
Confident
Excited
Enthusiastic
Powerful
Fantastic
Lucky
Hopeful
Content
Focused
Good
Grateful
Confused
Sad
Ashamed
Lonely
Frustrated
Angry
Hurt
Jealous
Exhausted
Overwhelmed
Tired
Scared

I Spent most of today with

____

____

____

____

What I like the most today

____

____

____

____

What I like the least today

____

____

____

____

TODAY'S CHOICES

Physically	Mentally	Spiritually
☐ working	☐ reading	☐ meditating
☐ exercising	☐ doing a project	☐ praying
☐ shopping	☐ practicing	☐ with nature
☐ gardening	☐ organizing	☐ being challenged
☐ traveling	☐ thinking	☐ with family + friends
☐ playing	☐ planning	☐ relaxing

More thoughts...etc.....

SMTWTFS _________________ 20___ ___ AM / PM

☐ Sunny ☐ partly cloudy ☐ cloudy ☐ rain ☐ Snow

-10 zero 10's 20's 30's 40's 50's 60's 70's 80's 90's 100's
☐ ☐ ☐ ☐ ☐ ☐ ☐ ☐ ☐ ☐ ☐ ☐

I FEEL
Happy
Confident
Excited
Enthusiastic
Powerful
Fantastic
Lucky
Hopeful
Content
Focused
Good
Grateful
Confused
Sad
Ashamed
Lonely
Frustrated
Angry
Hurt
Jealous
Exhausted
Overwhelmed
Tired
Scared

I Spent most of today with

____
____
____
____
____

What I like the most today

____
____
____
____

What I like the least today

____
____
____

TODAY'S CHOICES

Physically	Mentally	Spiritually
☐ working	☐ reading	☐ meditating
☐ exercising	☐ doing a project	☐ praying
☐ shopping	☐ practicing	☐ with nature
☐ gardening	☐ organizing	☐ being challenged
☐ traveling	☐ thinking	☐ with family + friends
☐ playing	☐ planning	☐ relaxing

More thoughts...etc.....

SMTWTFS _________________________ 20 ___ ___ AM / PM

☐ Sunny ☐ partly cloudy ☐ cloudy ☐ rain ☐ Snow

-10 zero 10's 20's 30's 40's 50's 60's 70's 80's 90's 100's
☐   ☐   ☐   ☐   ☐   ☐   ☐   ☐   ☐   ☐   ☐   ☐

I FEEL
Happy
Confident
Excited
Enthusiastic
Powerful
Fantastic
Lucky
Hopeful
Content
Focused
Good
Grateful
Confused
Sad
Ashamed
Lonely
Frustrated
Angry
Hurt
Jealous
Exhausted
Overwhelmed
Tired
Scared

I Spent most of today with

____
____
____
____
____

What I like the most today

____
____
____
____

What I like the least today

____
____
____
____

TODAY'S CHOICES

Physically	Mentally	Spiritually
☐ working	☐ reading	☐ meditating
☐ exercising	☐ doing a project	☐ praying
☐ shopping	☐ practicing	☐ with nature
☐ gardening	☐ organizing	☐ being challenged
☐ traveling	☐ thinking	☐ with family + friends
☐ playing	☐ planning	☐ relaxing

More thoughts...etc.....

SMTWTFS _______________ 20___ ___
AM
PM

☐ Sunny   ☐ partly cloudy   ☐ cloudy   ☐ rain   ☐ Snow

-10   zero   10's   20's   30's   40's   50's   60's   70's   80's   90's   100's
☐   ☐   ☐   ☐   ☐   ☐   ☐   ☐   ☐   ☐   ☐   ☐

I FEEL
Happy
Confident
Excited
Enthusiastic
Powerful
Fantastic
Lucky
Hopeful
Content
Focused
Good
Grateful
Confused
Sad
Ashamed
Lonely
Frustrated
Angry
Hurt
Jealous
Exhausted
Overwhelmed
Tired
Scared

I Spent most of today with

What I like the most today

What I like the least today

TODAY'S CHOICES

Physically	Mentally	Spiritually
☐ working	☐ reading	☐ meditating
☐ exercising	☐ doing a project	☐ praying
☐ shopping	☐ practicing	☐ with nature
☐ gardening	☐ organizing	☐ being challenged
☐ traveling	☐ thinking	☐ with family + friends
☐ playing	☐ planning	☐ relaxing

More thoughts...etc.....

SMTWTFS _______________ 20 ___ ___ AM / PM

☐ Sunny   ☐ partly cloudy   ☐ cloudy   ☐ rain   ☐ Snow

-10 zero 10's 20's 30's 40's 50's 60's 70's 80's 90's 100's
☐   ☐   ☐   ☐   ☐   ☐   ☐   ☐   ☐   ☐   ☐   ☐

I FEEL
- Happy
- Confident
- Excited
- Enthusiastic
- Powerful
- Fantastic
- Lucky
- Hopeful
- Content
- Focused
- Good
- Grateful
- Confused
- Sad
- Ashamed
- Lonely
- Frustrated
- Angry
- Hurt
- Jealous
- Exhausted
- Overwhelmed
- Tired
- Scared

I Spent most of today with

____
____
____
____
____

What I like the most today

____
____
____
____

What I like the least today

____
____
____

TODAY'S CHOICES

Physically	Mentally	Spiritually
☐ working	☐ reading	☐ meditating
☐ exercising	☐ doing a project	☐ praying
☐ shopping	☐ practicing	☐ with nature
☐ gardening	☐ organizing	☐ being challenged
☐ traveling	☐ thinking	☐ with family + friends
☐ playing	☐ planning	☐ relaxing
__________	__________	__________
__________	__________	__________
__________	__________	__________

More thoughts...etc.....

____

____

____

____

SMTWTFS _________________ 20___ ___ AM / PM

□ Sunny □ partly cloudy □ cloudy □ rain □ Snow

-10 zero 10's 20's 30's 40's 50's 60's 70's 80's 90's 100's
□ □ □ □ □ □ □ □ □ □ □ □

I FEEL
- Happy
- Confident
- Excited
- Enthusiastic
- Powerful
- Fantastic
- Lucky
- Hopeful
- Content
- Focused
- Good
- Grateful
- Confused
- Sad
- Ashamed
- Lonely
- Frustrated
- Angry
- Hurt
- Jealous
- Exhausted
- Overwhelmed
- Tired
- Scared

I Spent most of today with

____
____
____
____
____

What I like the most today

____
____
____
____

What I like the least today

____
____
____
____

TODAY'S CHOICES

Physically	Mentally	Spiritually
☐ working	☐ reading	☐ meditating
☐ exercising	☐ doing a project	☐ praying
☐ shopping	☐ practicing	☐ with nature
☐ gardening	☐ organizing	☐ being challenged
☐ traveling	☐ thinking	☐ with family + friends
☐ playing	☐ planning	☐ relaxing

More thoughts...etc.....

SMTWTFS ________________________ 20___ ___ AM / PM

☐ Sunny   ☐ partly cloudy   ☐ cloudy   ☐ rain   ☐ Snow

-10 zero 10's 20's 30's 40's 50's 60's 70's 80's 90's 100's
☐   ☐   ☐   ☐   ☐   ☐   ☐   ☐   ☐   ☐   ☐   ☐

I FEEL
Happy
Confident
Excited
Enthusiastic
Powerful
Fantastic
Lucky
Hopeful
Content
Focused
Good
Grateful
Confused
Sad
Ashamed
Lonely
Frustrated
Angry
Hurt
Jealous
Exhausted
Overwhelmed
Tired
Scared

I Spent most of today with

____
____
____
____
____

What I like the most today

____
____
____
____

What I like the least today

____
____
____
____

TODAY'S CHOICES

Physically	Mentally	Spiritually
☐ working	☐ reading	☐ meditating
☐ exercising	☐ doing a project	☐ praying
☐ shopping	☐ practicing	☐ with nature
☐ gardening	☐ organizing	☐ being challenged
☐ traveling	☐ thinking	☐ with family + friends
☐ playing	☐ planning	☐ relaxing

More thoughts...etc.....

SMTWTFS _______________ 20___ ___
AM
PM

☐ Sunny   ☐ partly cloudy   ☐ cloudy   ☐ rain   ☐ Snow

-10   zero   10's   20's   30's   40's   50's   60's   70's   80's   90's   100's
☐   ☐   ☐   ☐   ☐   ☐   ☐   ☐   ☐   ☐   ☐   ☐

I FEEL
Happy
Confident
Excited
Enthusiastic
Powerful
Fantastic
Lucky
Hopeful
Content
Focused
Good
Grateful
Confused
Sad
Ashamed
Lonely
Frustrated
Angry
Hurt
Jealous
Exhausted
Overwhelmed
Tired
Scared

I Spent most of today with

What I like the most today

What I like the least today

TODAY'S CHOICES

Physically	Mentally	Spiritually
☐ working	☐ reading	☐ meditating
☐ exercising	☐ doing a project	☐ praying
☐ shopping	☐ practicing	☐ with nature
☐ gardening	☐ organizing	☐ being challenged
☐ traveling	☐ thinking	☐ with family + friends
☐ playing	☐ planning	☐ relaxing

More thoughts...etc.....

SMTWTFS ______________ 20___ ___ AM PM

☐ Sunny   ☐ partly cloudy   ☐ cloudy   ☐ rain   ☐ Snow

-10   zero   10's   20's   30's   40's   50's   60's   70's   80's   90's   100's
☐   ☐   ☐   ☐   ☐   ☐   ☐   ☐   ☐   ☐   ☐   ☐

I FEEL

Happy
Confident
Excited
Enthusiastic
Powerful
Fantastic
Lucky
Hopeful
Content
Focused
Good
Grateful
Confused
Sad
Ashamed
Lonely
Frustrated
Angry
Hurt
Jealous
Exhausted
Overwhelmed
Tired
Scared

I Spent most of today with

____
____
____
____
____

What I like the most today

____
____
____
____

What I like the least today

____
____
____

TODAY'S CHOICES

Physically	Mentally	Spiritually
☐ working	☐ reading	☐ meditating
☐ exercising	☐ doing a project	☐ praying
☐ shopping	☐ practicing	☐ with nature
☐ gardening	☐ organizing	☐ being challenged
☐ traveling	☐ thinking	☐ with family + friends
☐ playing	☐ planning	☐ relaxing

More thoughts...etc.....

SMTWTFS ________________ 20___ ___ AM / PM

☐ Sunny ☐ partly cloudy ☐ cloudy ☐ rain ☐ Snow

-10 zero 10's 20's 30's 40's 50's 60's 70's 80's 90's 100's
☐   ☐   ☐   ☐   ☐   ☐   ☐   ☐   ☐   ☐   ☐   ☐

I FEEL
Happy
Confident
Excited
Enthusiastic
Powerful
Fantastic
Lucky
Hopeful
Content
Focused
Good
Grateful
Confused
Sad
Ashamed
Lonely
Frustrated
Angry
Hurt
Jealous
Exhausted
Overwhelmed
Tired
Scared

I Spent most of today with

____
____
____
____
____

What I like the most today

____
____
____
____

What I like the least today

____
____
____
____

TODAY'S CHOICES

Physically	Mentally	Spiritually
☐ working	☐ reading	☐ meditating
☐ exercising	☐ doing a project	☐ praying
☐ shopping	☐ practicing	☐ with nature
☐ gardening	☐ organizing	☐ being challenged
☐ traveling	☐ thinking	☐ with family + friends
☐ playing	☐ planning	☐ relaxing

More thoughts...etc.....

SMTWTFS _______________ 20__ __ AM PM

☐ Sunny ☐ partly cloudy ☐ cloudy ☐ rain ☐ Snow

-10 zero 10's 20's 30's 40's 50's 60's 70's 80's 90's 100's
☐   ☐   ☐   ☐   ☐   ☐   ☐   ☐   ☐   ☐   ☐   ☐

I FEEL
Happy
Confident
Excited
Enthusiastic
Powerful
Fantastic
Lucky
Hopeful
Content
Focused
Good
Grateful
Confused
Sad
Ashamed
Lonely
Frustrated
Angry
Hurt
Jealous
Exhausted
Overwhelmed
Tired
Scared

I spent most of today with
____
____
____
____
____

What I like the most today
____
____
____
____

What I like the least today
____
____
____
____

TODAY'S CHOICES

Physically	Mentally	Spiritually
☐ working	☐ reading	☐ meditating
☐ exercising	☐ doing a project	☐ praying
☐ shopping	☐ practicing	☐ with nature
☐ gardening	☐ organizing	☐ being challenged
☐ traveling	☐ thinking	☐ with family + friends
☐ playing	☐ planning	☐ relaxing

More thoughts...etc.....

SMTWTFS _________________ 20___ ___ AM PM

☐ Sunny ☐ partly cloudy ☐ cloudy ☐ rain ☐ Snow

-10 zero 10's 20's 30's 40's 50's 60's 70's 80's 90's 100's
☐   ☐   ☐   ☐   ☐   ☐   ☐   ☐   ☐   ☐   ☐   ☐

I FEEL

Happy
Confident
Excited
Enthusiastic
Powerful
Fantastic
Lucky
Hopeful
Content
Focused
Good
Grateful
Confused
Sad
Ashamed
Lonely
Frustrated
Angry
Hurt
Jealous
Exhausted
Overwhelmed
Tired
Scared

I Spent most of today with

____

____

____

____

What I like the most today

____

____

____

____

What I like the least today

____

____

____

____

TODAY'S CHOICES

Physically	Mentally	Spiritually
☐ working	☐ reading	☐ meditating
☐ exercising	☐ doing a project	☐ praying
☐ shopping	☐ practicing	☐ with nature
☐ gardening	☐ organizing	☐ being challenged
☐ traveling	☐ thinking	☐ with family + friends
☐ playing	☐ planning	☐ relaxing

More thoughts...etc.....

SMTWTFS _________________ 20___ ___ AM PM

☐ Sunny ☐ partly cloudy ☐ cloudy ☐ rain ☐ Snow

-10 zero 10's 20's 30's 40's 50's 60's 70's 80's 90's 100's
☐ ☐ ☐ ☐ ☐ ☐ ☐ ☐ ☐ ☐ ☐ ☐

I FEEL

| Happy |
| Confident |
| Excited |
| Enthusiastic |
| Powerful |
| Fantastic |
| Lucky |
| Hopeful |
| Content |
| Focused |
| Good |
| Grateful |
| Confused |
| Sad |
| Ashamed |
| Lonely |
| Frustrated |
| Angry |
| Hurt |
| Jealous |
| Exhausted |
| Overwhelmed |
| Tired |
| Scared |

I Spent most of today with

____
____
____
____
____

What I like the most today

____
____
____
____

What I like the least today

____
____
____
____

TODAY'S CHOICES

Physically	Mentally	Spiritually
☐ working	☐ reading	☐ meditating
☐ exercising	☐ doing a project	☐ praying
☐ shopping	☐ practicing	☐ with nature
☐ gardening	☐ organizing	☐ being challenged
☐ traveling	☐ thinking	☐ with family + friends
☐ playing	☐ planning	☐ relaxing

More thoughts...etc.....

SMTWTFS _______________ 20 ___ ___ AM PM

☐ Sunny ☐ partly cloudy ☐ cloudy ☐ rain ☐ Snow

-10 zero 10's 20's 30's 40's 50's 60's 70's 80's 90's 100's
☐   ☐   ☐   ☐   ☐   ☐   ☐   ☐   ☐   ☐   ☐   ☐

I FEEL
Happy
Confident
Excited
Enthusiastic
Powerful
Fantastic
Lucky
Hopeful
Content
Focused
Good
Grateful
Confused
Sad
Ashamed
Lonely
Frustrated
Angry
Hurt
Jealous
Exhausted
Overwhelmed
Tired
Scared

I Spent most of today with
____
____
____
____
____

What I like the most today
____
____
____
____

What I like the least today
____
____
____
____

TODAY'S CHOICES

Physically	Mentally	Spiritually
☐ working	☐ reading	☐ meditating
☐ exercising	☐ doing a project	☐ praying
☐ shopping	☐ practicing	☐ with nature
☐ gardening	☐ organizing	☐ being challenged
☐ traveling	☐ thinking	☐ with family + friends
☐ playing	☐ planning	☐ relaxing

More thoughts...etc.....

SMTWTFS _______________________ 20___ ___ AM PM

□ Sunny   □ partly cloudy   □ cloudy   □ rain   □ Snow

-10 zero 10's 20's 30's 40's 50's 60's 70's 80's 90's 100's
□   □   □   □   □   □   □   □   □   □   □   □

I FEEL

Happy
Confident
Excited
Enthusiastic
Powerful
Fantastic
Lucky
Hopeful
Content
Focused
Good
Grateful
Confused
Sad
Ashamed
Lonely
Frustrated
Angry
Hurt
Jealous
Exhausted
Overwhelmed
Tired
Scared

I Spent most of today with

____
____
____
____
____

What I like the most today

____
____
____
____

What I like the least today

____
____
____
____

TODAY'S CHOICES

Physically	Mentally	Spiritually
☐ working	☐ reading	☐ meditating
☐ exercising	☐ doing a project	☐ praying
☐ shopping	☐ practicing	☐ with nature
☐ gardening	☐ organizing	☐ being challenged
☐ traveling	☐ thinking	☐ with family + friends
☐ playing	☐ planning	☐ relaxing

More thoughts...etc.....

SMTWTFS _________________ 20___ ___ AM PM

☐ Sunny   ☐ partly cloudy   ☐ cloudy   ☐ rain   ☐ Snow

-10 zero 10's 20's 30's 40's 50's 60's 70's 80's 90's 100's
☐   ☐   ☐   ☐   ☐   ☐   ☐   ☐   ☐   ☐   ☐   ☐

I FEEL

Happy
Confident
Excited
Enthusiastic
Powerful
Fantastic
Lucky
Hopeful
Content
Focused
Good
Grateful
Confused
Sad
Ashamed
Lonely
Frustrated
Angry
Hurt
Jealous
Exhausted
Overwhelmed
Tired
Scared

I spent most of today with
____
____
____
____
____

What I like the most today
____
____
____
____
____

What I like the least today
____
____
____
____
____

TODAY'S CHOICES

Physically	Mentally	Spiritually
☐ working	☐ reading	☐ meditating
☐ exercising	☐ doing a project	☐ praying
☐ shopping	☐ practicing	☐ with nature
☐ gardening	☐ organizing	☐ being challenged
☐ traveling	☐ thinking	☐ with family + friends
☐ playing	☐ planning	☐ relaxing

More thoughts...etc.....

SMTWTFS _________________ 20___ ___ AM / PM

☐ Sunny   ☐ partly cloudy   ☐ cloudy   ☐ rain   ☐ Snow

-10 zero 10's 20's 30's 40's 50's 60's 70's 80's 90's 100's
☐   ☐   ☐   ☐   ☐   ☐   ☐   ☐   ☐   ☐   ☐   ☐

I FEEL

- Happy
- Confident
- Excited
- Enthusiastic
- Powerful
- Fantastic
- Lucky
- Hopeful
- Content
- Focused
- Good
- Grateful
- Confused
- Sad
- Ashamed
- Lonely
- Frustrated
- Angry
- Hurt
- Jealous
- Exhausted
- Overwhelmed
- Tired
- Scared

I Spent most of today with

____
____
____
____
____

What I like the most today

____
____
____
____
____

What I like the least today

____
____
____
____

TODAY'S CHOICES

Physically	Mentally	Spiritually
☐ working	☐ reading	☐ meditating
☐ exercising	☐ doing a project	☐ praying
☐ shopping	☐ practicing	☐ with nature
☐ gardening	☐ organizing	☐ being challenged
☐ traveling	☐ thinking	☐ with family + friends
☐ playing	☐ planning	☐ relaxing

More thoughts...etc.....

SMTWTFS _________________ 20___ ___

AM
PM

☐ Sunny ☐ partly cloudy ☐ cloudy ☐ rain ☐ Snow

-10 zero 10's 20's 30's 40's 50's 60's 70's 80's 90's 100's
☐   ☐   ☐   ☐   ☐   ☐   ☐   ☐   ☐   ☐   ☐   ☐

I FEEL
Happy
Confident
Excited
Enthusiastic
Powerful
Fantastic
Lucky
Hopeful
Content
Focused
Good
Grateful
Confused
Sad
Ashamed
Lonely
Frustrated
Angry
Hurt
Jealous
Exhausted
Overwhelmed
Tired
Scared

I Spent most of today with

____
____
____
____
____

What I like the most today

____
____
____
____

What I like the least today

____
____
____
____

TODAY'S CHOICES

Physically	Mentally	Spiritually
☐ working	☐ reading	☐ meditating
☐ exercising	☐ doing a project	☐ praying
☐ shopping	☐ practicing	☐ with nature
☐ gardening	☐ organizing	☐ being challenged
☐ traveling	☐ thinking	☐ with family + friends
☐ playing	☐ planning	☐ relaxing

More thoughts...etc.....

SMTWTFS _________________ 20___ ___ AM PM

☐ Sunny ☐ partly cloudy ☐ cloudy ☐ rain ☐ Snow

-10 zero 10's 20's 30's 40's 50's 60's 70's 80's 90's 100's
☐   ☐   ☐   ☐   ☐   ☐   ☐   ☐   ☐   ☐   ☐   ☐

I FEEL
Happy
Confident
Excited
Enthusiastic
Powerful
Fantastic
Lucky
Hopeful
Content
Focused
Good
Grateful
Confused
Sad
Ashamed
Lonely
Frustrated
Angry
Hurt
Jealous
Exhausted
Overwhelmed
Tired
Scared

I Spent most of today with

____
____
____
____
____

What I like the most today

____
____
____
____

What I like the least today

____
____
____

TODAY'S CHOICES

Physically	Mentally	Spiritually
☐ working	☐ reading	☐ meditating
☐ exercising	☐ doing a project	☐ praying
☐ shopping	☐ practicing	☐ with nature
☐ gardening	☐ organizing	☐ being challenged
☐ traveling	☐ thinking	☐ with family + friends
☐ playing	☐ planning	☐ relaxing

More thoughts...etc.....

SMTWTFS _______________ 20__ __ AM PM

☐ Sunny ☐ partly cloudy ☐ cloudy ☐ rain ☐ Snow

-10 zero 10's 20's 30's 40's 50's 60's 70's 80's 90's 100's
☐ ☐ ☐ ☐ ☐ ☐ ☐ ☐ ☐ ☐ ☐ ☐

I FEEL
- Happy
- Confident
- Excited
- Enthusiastic
- Powerful
- Fantastic
- Lucky
- Hopeful
- Content
- Focused
- Good
- Grateful
- Confused
- Sad
- Ashamed
- Lonely
- Frustrated
- Angry
- Hurt
- Jealous
- Exhausted
- Overwhelmed
- Tired
- Scared

I Spent most of today with

____
____
____
____
____

What I like the most today

____
____
____
____

What I like the least today

____
____
____

TODAY'S CHOICES

Physically	Mentally	Spiritually
☐ working	☐ reading	☐ meditating
☐ exercising	☐ doing a project	☐ praying
☐ shopping	☐ practicing	☐ with nature
☐ gardening	☐ organizing	☐ being challenged
☐ traveling	☐ thinking	☐ with family + friends
☐ playing	☐ planning	☐ relaxing

More thoughts...etc.....

SMTWTFS _________________ 20___ ___ AM / PM

☀ ☐ Sunny   ⛅ ☐ partly cloudy   ☁ ☐ cloudy   🌧 ☐ rain   ❄ ☐ Snow

-10   zero   10's   20's   30's   40's   50's   60's   70's   80's   90's   100's
☐   ☐   ☐   ☐   ☐   ☐   ☐   ☐   ☐   ☐   ☐   ☐

I FEEL
Happy
Confident
Excited
Enthusiastic
Powerful
Fantastic
Lucky
Hopeful
Content
Focused
Good
Grateful
Confused
Sad
Ashamed
Lonely
Frustrated
Angry
Hurt
Jealous
Exhausted
Overwhelmed
Tired
Scared

I Spent most of today with

____
____
____
____
____

What I like the most today

____
____
____
____

What I like the least today

____
____
____
____

TODAY'S CHOICES

Physically	Mentally	Spiritually
☐ working	☐ reading	☐ meditating
☐ exercising	☐ doing a project	☐ praying
☐ shopping	☐ practicing	☐ with nature
☐ gardening	☐ organizing	☐ being challenged
☐ traveling	☐ thinking	☐ with family + friends
☐ playing	☐ planning	☐ relaxing

More thoughts...etc.....

SMTWTFS _________________ 20 ___ ___

AM
PM

☐ Sunny   ☐ partly cloudy   ☐ cloudy   ☐ rain   ☐ Snow

-10   zero   10's   20's   30's   40's   50's   60's   70's   80's   90's   100's
☐   ☐   ☐   ☐   ☐   ☐   ☐   ☐   ☐   ☐   ☐   ☐

I FEEL

Happy
Confident
Excited
Enthusiastic
Powerful
Fantastic
Lucky
Hopeful
Content
Focused
Good
Grateful
Confused
Sad
Ashamed
Lonely
Frustrated
Angry
Hurt
Jealous
Exhausted
Overwhelmed
Tired
Scared

I Spent most of today with

____

____

____

____

What I like the most today

____

____

____

____

What I like the least today

____

____

____

____

TODAY'S CHOICES

Physically	Mentally	Spiritually
☐ working	☐ reading	☐ meditating
☐ exercising	☐ doing a project	☐ praying
☐ shopping	☐ practicing	☐ with nature
☐ gardening	☐ organizing	☐ being challenged
☐ traveling	☐ thinking	☐ with family + friends
☐ playing	☐ planning	☐ relaxing

More thoughts...etc.....

SMTWTFS _________________ 20 ___ ___ AM PM

☐ Sunny   ☐ partly cloudy   ☐ cloudy   ☐ rain   ☐ Snow

-10 zero 10's 20's 30's 40's 50's 60's 70's 80's 90's 100's
☐   ☐   ☐   ☐   ☐   ☐   ☐   ☐   ☐   ☐   ☐   ☐

I FEEL
Happy
Confident
Excited
Enthusiastic
Powerful
Fantastic
Lucky
Hopeful
Content
Focused
Good
Grateful
Confused
Sad
Ashamed
Lonely
Frustrated
Angry
Hurt
Jealous
Exhausted
Overwhelmed
Tired
Scared

I Spent most of today with

____

____

____

____

____

What I like the most today

____

____

____

____

What I like the least today

____

____

____

____

TODAY'S CHOICES

Physically	Mentally	Spiritually
☐ working	☐ reading	☐ meditating
☐ exercising	☐ doing a project	☐ praying
☐ shopping	☐ practicing	☐ with nature
☐ gardening	☐ organizing	☐ being challenged
☐ traveling	☐ thinking	☐ with family + friends
☐ playing	☐ planning	☐ relaxing

More thoughts...etc.....

SMTWTFS _______________ 20___ ___
AM
PM

☐ Sunny   ☐ partly cloudy   ☐ cloudy   ☐ rain   ☐ Snow

-10   zero   10's   20's   30's   40's   50's   60's   70's   80's   90's   100's
☐   ☐   ☐   ☐   ☐   ☐   ☐   ☐   ☐   ☐   ☐   ☐

I FEEL
Happy
Confident
Excited
Enthusiastic
Powerful
Fantastic
Lucky
Hopeful
Content
Focused
Good
Grateful
Confused
Sad
Ashamed
Lonely
Frustrated
Angry
Hurt
Jealous
Exhausted
Overwhelmed
Tired
Scared

I spent most of today with
____
____
____
____
____

What I like the most today
____
____
____
____

What I like the least today
____
____
____
____

TODAY'S CHOICES

Physically	Mentally	Spiritually
☐ working	☐ reading	☐ meditating
☐ exercising	☐ doing a project	☐ praying
☐ shopping	☐ practicing	☐ with nature
☐ gardening	☐ organizing	☐ being challenged
☐ traveling	☐ thinking	☐ with family + friends
☐ playing	☐ planning	☐ relaxing

More thoughts...etc.....

SMTWTFS _________________ 20 ___ ___ AM PM

□ Sunny □ partly cloudy □ cloudy □ rain □ Snow

-10 zero 10's 20's 30's 40's 50's 60's 70's 80's 90's 100's
□   □   □   □   □   □   □   □   □   □   □   □

I FEEL
Happy
Confident
Excited
Enthusiastic
Powerful
Fantastic
Lucky
Hopeful
Content
Focused
Good
Grateful
Confused
Sad
Ashamed
Lonely
Frustrated
Angry
Hurt
Jealous
Exhausted
Overwhelmed
Tired
Scared

I Spent most of today with

____
____
____
____
____

What I like the most today

____
____
____
____

What I like the least today

____
____
____
____

TODAY'S CHOICES

Physically	Mentally	Spiritually
☐ working	☐ reading	☐ meditating
☐ exercising	☐ doing a project	☐ praying
☐ shopping	☐ practicing	☐ with nature
☐ gardening	☐ organizing	☐ being challenged
☐ traveling	☐ thinking	☐ with family + friends
☐ playing	☐ planning	☐ relaxing

More thoughts...etc.....

SMTWTFS _________________ 20___ ___ AM / PM

☐ Sunny ☐ partly cloudy ☐ cloudy ☐ rain ☐ Snow

-10 zero 10's 20's 30's 40's 50's 60's 70's 80's 90's 100's
☐   ☐   ☐   ☐   ☐   ☐   ☐   ☐   ☐   ☐   ☐   ☐

I FEEL
Happy
Confident
Excited
Enthusiastic
Powerful
Fantastic
Lucky
Hopeful
Content
Focused
Good
Grateful
Confused
Sad
Ashamed
Lonely
Frustrated
Angry
Hurt
Jealous
Exhausted
Overwhelmed
Tired
Scared

I Spent most of today with
____
____
____
____
____

What I like the most today
____
____
____
____

What I like the least today
____
____
____
____

TODAY'S CHOICES

Physically	Mentally	Spiritually
☐ working	☐ reading	☐ meditating
☐ exercising	☐ doing a project	☐ praying
☐ shopping	☐ practicing	☐ with nature
☐ gardening	☐ organizing	☐ being challenged
☐ traveling	☐ thinking	☐ with family + friends
☐ playing	☐ planning	☐ relaxing

More thoughts...etc.....

SMTWTFS _________________ 20___ ___ AM PM

☀
☐ Sunny   ☐ partly cloudy   ☐ cloudy   ☐ rain   ☐ Snow

-10   zero   10's   20's   30's   40's   50's   60's   70's   80's   90's   100's
☐   ☐   ☐   ☐   ☐   ☐   ☐   ☐   ☐   ☐   ☐   ☐

I FEEL
Happy
Confident
Excited
Enthusiastic
Powerful
Fantastic
Lucky
Hopeful
Content
Focused
Good
Grateful
Confused
Sad
Ashamed
Lonely
Frustrated
Angry
Hurt
Jealous
Exhausted
Overwhelmed
Tired
Scared

I Spent most of today with

____

____

____

____

____

What I like the most today

____

____

____

____

____

What I like the least today

____

____

____

TODAY'S CHOICES

Physically	Mentally	Spiritually
☐ working	☐ reading	☐ meditating
☐ exercising	☐ doing a project	☐ praying
☐ shopping	☐ practicing	☐ with nature
☐ gardening	☐ organizing	☐ being challenged
☐ traveling	☐ thinking	☐ with family + friends
☐ playing	☐ planning	☐ relaxing

More thoughts...etc.....

S M T W T F S _______________ 20___ ___

AM
PM

☐ Sunny   ☐ partly cloudy   ☐ cloudy   ☐ rain   ☐ Snow

-10 zero 10's 20's 30's 40's 50's 60's 70's 80's 90's 100's
☐   ☐   ☐   ☐   ☐   ☐   ☐   ☐   ☐   ☐   ☐   ☐

I FEEL
Happy
Confident
Excited
Enthusiastic
Powerful
Fantastic
Lucky
Hopeful
Content
Focused
Good
Grateful
Confused
Sad
Ashamed
Lonely
Frustrated
Angry
Hurt
Jealous
Exhausted
Overwhelmed
Tired
Scared

I Spent most of today with

____
____
____
____
____

What I like the most today

____
____
____
____

What I like the least today

____
____
____

TODAY'S CHOICES

Physically	Mentally	Spiritually
☐ working	☐ reading	☐ meditating
☐ exercising	☐ doing a project	☐ praying
☐ shopping	☐ practicing	☐ with nature
☐ gardening	☐ organizing	☐ being challenged
☐ traveling	☐ thinking	☐ with family + friends
☐ playing	☐ planning	☐ relaxing

More thoughts...etc.....

SMTWTFS _______________ 20___ ___ AM / PM

☐ Sunny ☐ partly cloudy ☐ cloudy ☐ rain ☐ Snow

-10 zero 10's 20's 30's 40's 50's 60's 70's 80's 90's 100's
☐ ☐ ☐ ☐ ☐ ☐ ☐ ☐ ☐ ☐ ☐ ☐

I FEEL
Happy
Confident
Excited
Enthusiastic
Powerful
Fantastic
Lucky
Hopeful
Content
Focused
Good
Grateful
Confused
Sad
Ashamed
Lonely
Frustrated
Angry
Hurt
Jealous
Exhausted
Overwhelmed
Tired
Scared

I Spent most of today with

____
____
____
____
____

What I like the most today

____
____
____
____

What I like the least today

____
____
____
____

TODAY'S CHOICES

Physically	Mentally	Spiritually
☐ working	☐ reading	☐ meditating
☐ exercising	☐ doing a project	☐ praying
☐ shopping	☐ practicing	☐ with nature
☐ gardening	☐ organizing	☐ being challenged
☐ traveling	☐ thinking	☐ with family + friends
☐ playing	☐ planning	☐ relaxing

More thoughts...etc.....

SMTWTFS _________________ 20___ ___

AM
PM

☐ Sunny ☐ partly cloudy ☐ cloudy ☐ rain ☐ Snow

-10 zero 10's 20's 30's 40's 50's 60's 70's 80's 90's 100's
☐   ☐   ☐   ☐   ☐   ☐   ☐   ☐   ☐   ☐   ☐   ☐

I FEEL
Happy
Confident
Excited
Enthusiastic
Powerful
Fantastic
Lucky
Hopeful
Content
Focused
Good
Grateful
Confused
Sad
Ashamed
Lonely
Frustrated
Angry
Hurt
Jealous
Exhausted
Overwhelmed
Tired
Scared

I Spent most of today with

____
____
____
____
____

What I like the most today

____
____
____
____

What I like the least today

____
____
____

TODAY'S CHOICES

Physically	Mentally	Spiritually
☐ working	☐ reading	☐ meditating
☐ exercising	☐ doing a project	☐ praying
☐ shopping	☐ practicing	☐ with nature
☐ gardening	☐ organizing	☐ being challenged
☐ traveling	☐ thinking	☐ with family + friends
☐ playing	☐ planning	☐ relaxing

More thoughts...etc.....

SMTWTFS _______________ 20___ ___ AM / PM

☐ Sunny   ☐ partly cloudy   ☐ cloudy   ☐ rain   ☐ Snow

-10   zero   10's   20's   30's   40's   50's   60's   70's   80's   90's   100's
☐   ☐   ☐   ☐   ☐   ☐   ☐   ☐   ☐   ☐   ☐   ☐

I FEEL
Happy
Confident
Excited
Enthusiastic
Powerful
Fantastic
Lucky
Hopeful
Content
Focused
Good
Grateful
Confused
Sad
Ashamed
Lonely
Frustrated
Angry
Hurt
Jealous
Exhausted
Overwhelmed
Tired
Scared

I Spent most of today with

____
____
____
____
____

What I like the most today

____
____
____
____

What I like the least today

____
____
____

TODAY'S CHOICES

Physically	Mentally	Spiritually
☐ working	☐ reading	☐ meditating
☐ exercising	☐ doing a project	☐ praying
☐ shopping	☐ practicing	☐ with nature
☐ gardening	☐ organizing	☐ being challenged
☐ traveling	☐ thinking	☐ with family + friends
☐ playing	☐ planning	☐ relaxing

More thoughts...etc.....

SMTWTFS _______________ 20___ ___ AM PM

☐ Sunny   ☐ partly cloudy   ☐ cloudy   ☐ rain   ☐ Snow

-10 zero 10's 20's 30's 40's 50's 60's 70's 80's 90's 100's
☐   ☐   ☐   ☐   ☐   ☐   ☐   ☐   ☐   ☐   ☐   ☐

I FEEL
Happy
Confident
Excited
Enthusiastic
Powerful
Fantastic
Lucky
Hopeful
Content
Focused
Good
Grateful
Confused
Sad
Ashamed
Lonely
Frustrated
Angry
Hurt
Jealous
Exhausted
Overwhelmed
Tired
Scared

I Spent most of today with
____
____
____
____
____

What I like the most today
____
____
____
____

What I like the least today
____
____
____

TODAY'S CHOICES

Physically	Mentally	Spiritually
☐ working	☐ reading	☐ meditating
☐ exercising	☐ doing a project	☐ praying
☐ shopping	☐ practicing	☐ with nature
☐ gardening	☐ organizing	☐ being challenged
☐ traveling	☐ thinking	☐ with family + friends
☐ playing	☐ planning	☐ relaxing

More thoughts...etc.....

SMTWTFS _____________ 20___ ___

AM
PM

☐ Sunny   ☐ partly cloudy   ☐ cloudy   ☐ rain   ☐ Snow

-10	zero	10's	20's	30's	40's	50's	60's	70's	80's	90's	100's
☐	☐	☐	☐	☐	☐	☐	☐	☐	☐	☐	☐

I FEEL

- Happy
- Confident
- Excited
- Enthusiastic
- Powerful
- Fantastic
- Lucky
- Hopeful
- Content
- Focused
- Good
- Grateful
- Confused
- Sad
- Ashamed
- Lonely
- Frustrated
- Angry
- Hurt
- Jealous
- Exhausted
- Overwhelmed
- Tired
- Scared

I Spent most of today with

____

____

____

____

____

What I like the most today

____

____

____

____

What I like the least today

____

____

____

____

TODAY'S CHOICES

Physically	Mentally	Spiritually
☐ working	☐ reading	☐ meditating
☐ exercising	☐ doing a project	☐ praying
☐ shopping	☐ practicing	☐ with nature
☐ gardening	☐ organizing	☐ being challenged
☐ traveling	☐ thinking	☐ with family + friends
☐ playing	☐ planning	☐ relaxing

More thoughts...etc.....

SMTWTFS _______________ 20___ ___

AM
PM

☐ Sunny   ☐ partly cloudy   ☐ cloudy   ☐ rain   ☐ Snow

-10   zero   10's   20's   30's   40's   50's   60's   70's   80's   90's   100's
☐   ☐   ☐   ☐   ☐   ☐   ☐   ☐   ☐   ☐   ☐   ☐

I FEEL
Happy
Confident
Excited
Enthusiastic
Powerful
Fantastic
Lucky
Hopeful
Content
Focused
Good
Grateful
Confused
Sad
Ashamed
Lonely
Frustrated
Angry
Hurt
Jealous
Exhausted
Overwhelmed
Tired
Scared

I Spent most of today with

____

____

____

____

____

What I like the most today

____

____

____

____

What I like the least today

____

____

____

____

TODAY'S CHOICES

Physically	Mentally	Spiritually
☐ working	☐ reading	☐ meditating
☐ exercising	☐ doing a project	☐ praying
☐ shopping	☐ practicing	☐ with nature
☐ gardening	☐ organizing	☐ being challenged
☐ traveling	☐ thinking	☐ with family + friends
☐ playing	☐ planning	☐ relaxing

More thoughts...etc.....

SMTWTFS _________________________ 20___ ___ AM / PM

☐ Sunny ☐ partly cloudy ☐ cloudy ☐ rain ☐ Snow

-10 zero 10's 20's 30's 40's 50's 60's 70's 80's 90's 100's
☐   ☐   ☐   ☐   ☐   ☐   ☐   ☐   ☐   ☐   ☐   ☐

I FEEL
- Happy
- Confident
- Excited
- Enthusiastic
- Powerful
- Fantastic
- Lucky
- Hopeful
- Content
- Focused
- Good
- Grateful
- Confused
- Sad
- Ashamed
- Lonely
- Frustrated
- Angry
- Hurt
- Jealous
- Exhausted
- Overwhelmed
- Tired
- Scared

I Spent most of today with

____

____

____

____

____

What I like the most today

____

____

____

____

What I like the least today

____

____

____

TODAY'S CHOICES

Physically	Mentally	Spiritually
☐ working	☐ reading	☐ meditating
☐ exercising	☐ doing a project	☐ praying
☐ shopping	☐ practicing	☐ with nature
☐ gardening	☐ organizing	☐ being challenged
☐ traveling	☐ thinking	☐ with family + friends
☐ playing	☐ planning	☐ relaxing

More thoughts...etc.....

SMTWTFS _________________ 20___ ___ AM PM

☐ Sunny ☐ partly cloudy ☐ cloudy ☐ rain ☐ Snow

-10 zero 10's 20's 30's 40's 50's 60's 70's 80's 90's 100's
☐   ☐   ☐   ☐   ☐   ☐   ☐   ☐   ☐   ☐   ☐   ☐

I FEEL
Happy
Confident
Excited
Enthusiastic
Powerful
Fantastic
Lucky
Hopeful
Content
Focused
Good
Grateful
Confused
Sad
Ashamed
Lonely
Frustrated
Angry
Hurt
Jealous
Exhausted
Overwhelmed
Tired
Scared

I Spent most of today with

____
____
____
____

What I like the most today

____
____
____
____

What I like the least today

____
____
____

TODAY'S CHOICES

Physically	Mentally	Spiritually
☐ working	☐ reading	☐ meditating
☐ exercising	☐ doing a project	☐ praying
☐ shopping	☐ practicing	☐ with nature
☐ gardening	☐ organizing	☐ being challenged
☐ traveling	☐ thinking	☐ with family + friends
☐ playing	☐ planning	☐ relaxing

More thoughts...etc.....

SMTWTFS _________________ 20___ ___ AM / PM

☐ Sunny   ☐ partly cloudy   ☐ cloudy   ☐ rain   ☐ Snow

-10 zero 10's 20's 30's 40's 50's 60's 70's 80's 90's 100's
☐   ☐   ☐   ☐   ☐   ☐   ☐   ☐   ☐   ☐   ☐   ☐

I FEEL
- Happy
- Confident
- Excited
- Enthusiastic
- Powerful
- Fantastic
- Lucky
- Hopeful
- Content
- Focused
- Good
- Grateful
- Confused
- Sad
- Ashamed
- Lonely
- Frustrated
- Angry
- Hurt
- Jealous
- Exhausted
- Overwhelmed
- Tired
- Scared

I Spent most of today with

____
____
____
____
____

What I like the most today

____
____
____
____

What I like the least today

____
____
____

TODAY'S CHOICES

Physically	Mentally	Spiritually
☐ working	☐ reading	☐ meditating
☐ exercising	☐ doing a project	☐ praying
☐ shopping	☐ practicing	☐ with nature
☐ gardening	☐ organizing	☐ being challenged
☐ traveling	☐ thinking	☐ with family + friends
☐ playing	☐ planning	☐ relaxing

More thoughts...etc.....

SMTWTFS _________________ 20__ __ AM / PM

☐ Sunny ☐ partly cloudy ☐ cloudy ☐ rain ☐ Snow

-10 zero 10's 20's 30's 40's 50's 60's 70's 80's 90's 100's
☐   ☐   ☐   ☐   ☐   ☐   ☐   ☐   ☐   ☐   ☐   ☐

I FEEL
- Happy
- Confident
- Excited
- Enthusiastic
- Powerful
- Fantastic
- Lucky
- Hopeful
- Content
- Focused
- Good
- Grateful
- Confused
- Sad
- Ashamed
- Lonely
- Frustrated
- Angry
- Hurt
- Jealous
- Exhausted
- Overwhelmed
- Tired
- Scared

I Spent most of today with

____
____
____
____

What I like the most today

____
____
____
____

What I like the least today

____
____
____
____

TODAY'S CHOICES

Physically	Mentally	Spiritually
☐ working	☐ reading	☐ meditating
☐ exercising	☐ doing a project	☐ praying
☐ shopping	☐ practicing	☐ with nature
☐ gardening	☐ organizing	☐ being challenged
☐ traveling	☐ thinking	☐ with family + friends
☐ playing	☐ planning	☐ relaxing

More thoughts...etc.....

SMTWTFS _________________ 20 ___ ___ AM PM

☐ Sunny ☐ partly cloudy ☐ cloudy ☐ rain ☐ Snow

-10 zero 10's 20's 30's 40's 50's 60's 70's 80's 90's 100's
☐   ☐   ☐   ☐   ☐   ☐   ☐   ☐   ☐   ☐   ☐   ☐

I FEEL
Happy
Confident
Excited
Enthusiastic
Powerful
Fantastic
Lucky
Hopeful
Content
Focused
Good
Grateful
Confused
Sad
Ashamed
Lonely
Frustrated
Angry
Hurt
Jealous
Exhausted
Overwhelmed
Tired
Scared

I Spent most of today with

____
____
____
____
____

What I like the most today

____
____
____
____

What I like the least today

____
____
____

TODAY'S CHOICES

Physically	Mentally	Spiritually
☐ working	☐ reading	☐ meditating
☐ exercising	☐ doing a project	☐ praying
☐ shopping	☐ practicing	☐ with nature
☐ gardening	☐ organizing	☐ being challenged
☐ traveling	☐ thinking	☐ with family + friends
☐ playing	☐ planning	☐ relaxing

_______________   _______________   _______________

_______________   _______________   _______________

_______________   _______________   _______________

More thoughts...etc.....

____

____

____

____

SMTWTFS _________________ 20___ ___ AM / PM

☐ Sunny ☐ partly cloudy ☐ cloudy ☐ rain ☐ Snow

-10 zero 10's 20's 30's 40's 50's 60's 70's 80's 90's 100's
☐ ☐ ☐ ☐ ☐ ☐ ☐ ☐ ☐ ☐ ☐ ☐

I FEEL

Happy
Confident
Excited
Enthusiastic
Powerful
Fantastic
Lucky
Hopeful
Content
Focused
Good
Grateful
Confused
Sad
Ashamed
Lonely
Frustrated
Angry
Hurt
Jealous
Exhausted
Overwhelmed
Tired
Scared

I Spent most of today with
____
____
____
____
____

What I like the most today
____
____
____
____

What I like the least today
____
____
____

TODAY'S CHOICES

Physically	Mentally	Spiritually
☐ working	☐ reading	☐ meditating
☐ exercising	☐ doing a project	☐ praying
☐ shopping	☐ practicing	☐ with nature
☐ gardening	☐ organizing	☐ being challenged
☐ traveling	☐ thinking	☐ with family + friends
☐ playing	☐ planning	☐ relaxing

More thoughts...etc.....

SMTWTFS ____________ 20__ __ AM PM

☐ Sunny ☐ partly cloudy ☐ cloudy ☐ rain ☐ Snow

-10 zero 10's 20's 30's 40's 50's 60's 70's 80's 90's 100's
☐ ☐ ☐ ☐ ☐ ☐ ☐ ☐ ☐ ☐ ☐ ☐

I FEEL
- Happy
- Confident
- Excited
- Enthusiastic
- Powerful
- Fantastic
- Lucky
- Hopeful
- Content
- Focused
- Good
- Grateful
- Confused
- Sad
- Ashamed
- Lonely
- Frustrated
- Angry
- Hurt
- Jealous
- Exhausted
- Overwhelmed
- Tired
- Scared

I Spent most of today with

____
____
____
____

What I like the most today

____
____
____

What I like the least today

____
____
____

TODAY'S CHOICES

Physically	Mentally	Spiritually
☐ working	☐ reading	☐ meditating
☐ exercising	☐ doing a project	☐ praying
☐ shopping	☐ practicing	☐ with nature
☐ gardening	☐ organizing	☐ being challenged
☐ traveling	☐ thinking	☐ with family + friends
☐ playing	☐ planning	☐ relaxing

More thoughts...etc.....

SMTWTFS _________________ 20___ ___ AM PM

☐ Sunny ☐ partly cloudy ☐ cloudy ☐ rain ☐ Snow

-10 zero 10's 20's 30's 40's 50's 60's 70's 80's 90's 100's
☐   ☐   ☐   ☐   ☐   ☐   ☐   ☐   ☐   ☐   ☐   ☐

I FEEL

Happy
Confident
Excited
Enthusiastic
Powerful
Fantastic
Lucky
Hopeful
Content
Focused
Good
Grateful
Confused
Sad
Ashamed
Lonely
Frustrated
Angry
Hurt
Jealous
Exhausted
Overwhelmed
Tired
Scared

I Spent most of today with

____
____
____
____
____

What I like the most today

____
____
____
____

What I like the least today

____
____
____
____

TODAY'S CHOICES

Physically	Mentally	Spiritually
☐ working	☐ reading	☐ meditating
☐ exercising	☐ doing a project	☐ praying
☐ shopping	☐ practicing	☐ with nature
☐ gardening	☐ organizing	☐ being challenged
☐ traveling	☐ thinking	☐ with family + friends
☐ playing	☐ planning	☐ relaxing

More thoughts...etc.....

SMTWTFS _________________ 20___ ___ AM / PM

☐ Sunny ☐ partly cloudy ☐ cloudy ☐ rain ☐ Snow

-10 zero 10's 20's 30's 40's 50's 60's 70's 80's 90's 100's
☐   ☐   ☐   ☐   ☐   ☐   ☐   ☐   ☐   ☐   ☐   ☐

I FEEL
- Happy
- Confident
- Excited
- Enthusiastic
- Powerful
- Fantastic
- Lucky
- Hopeful
- Content
- Focused
- Good
- Grateful
- Confused
- Sad
- Ashamed
- Lonely
- Frustrated
- Angry
- Hurt
- Jealous
- Exhausted
- Overwhelmed
- Tired
- Scared

I Spent most of today with

____

____

____

____

____

What I like the most today

____

____

____

____

What I like the least today

____

____

____

____

TODAY'S CHOICES

Physically	Mentally	Spiritually
☐ working	☐ reading	☐ meditating
☐ exercising	☐ doing a project	☐ praying
☐ shopping	☐ practicing	☐ with nature
☐ gardening	☐ organizing	☐ being challenged
☐ traveling	☐ thinking	☐ with family + friends
☐ playing	☐ planning	☐ relaxing

More thoughts...etc.....

SMTWTFS ____________ 20__ __ AM PM

☐ Sunny ☐ partly cloudy ☐ cloudy ☐ rain ☐ Snow

-10 zero 10's 20's 30's 40's 50's 60's 70's 80's 90's 100's
☐   ☐   ☐   ☐   ☐   ☐   ☐   ☐   ☐   ☐   ☐   ☐

I FEEL
Happy
Confident
Excited
Enthusiastic
Powerful
Fantastic
Lucky
Hopeful
Content
Focused
Good
Grateful
Confused
Sad
Ashamed
Lonely
Frustrated
Angry
Hurt
Jealous
Exhausted
Overwhelmed
Tired
Scared

I Spent most of today with

____
____
____
____
____

What I like the most today

____
____
____
____

What I like the least today

____
____
____

TODAY'S CHOICES

Physically	Mentally	Spiritually
☐ working	☐ reading	☐ meditating
☐ exercising	☐ doing a project	☐ praying
☐ shopping	☐ practicing	☐ with nature
☐ gardening	☐ organizing	☐ being challenged
☐ traveling	☐ thinking	☐ with family + friends
☐ playing	☐ planning	☐ relaxing

More thoughts...etc.....

SMTWTFS _________________ 20___ ___ AM PM

☐ Sunny   ☐ partly cloudy   ☐ cloudy   ☐ rain   ☐ Snow

-10 zero 10's 20's 30's 40's 50's 60's 70's 80's 90's 100's
☐   ☐   ☐   ☐   ☐   ☐   ☐   ☐   ☐   ☐   ☐   ☐

I FEEL
Happy
Confident
Excited
Enthusiastic
Powerful
Fantastic
Lucky
Hopeful
Content
Focused
Good
Grateful
Confused
Sad
Ashamed
Lonely
Frustrated
Angry
Hurt
Jealous
Exhausted
Overwhelmed
Tired
Scared

I Spent most of today with

____
____
____
____
____

What I like the most today

____
____
____
____

What I like the least today

____
____
____

TODAY'S CHOICES

Physically	Mentally	Spiritually
☐ working	☐ reading	☐ meditating
☐ exercising	☐ doing a project	☐ praying
☐ shopping	☐ practicing	☐ with nature
☐ gardening	☐ organizing	☐ being challenged
☐ traveling	☐ thinking	☐ with family + friends
☐ playing	☐ planning	☐ relaxing

More thoughts...etc.....

SMTWTFS _______________ 20___ ___ AM PM

□ Sunny □ partly cloudy □ cloudy □ rain □ Snow

-10 zero 10's 20's 30's 40's 50's 60's 70's 80's 90's 100's
□   □   □   □   □   □   □   □   □   □   □   □

I FEEL

- Happy
- Confident
- Excited
- Enthusiastic
- Powerful
- Fantastic
- Lucky
- Hopeful
- Content
- Focused
- Good
- Grateful
- Confused
- Sad
- Ashamed
- Lonely
- Frustrated
- Angry
- Hurt
- Jealous
- Exhausted
- Overwhelmed
- Tired
- Scared

I Spent most of today with

____
____
____
____
____

What I like the most today

____
____
____
____

What I like the least today

____
____
____
____

TODAY'S CHOICES

Physically	Mentally	Spiritually
☐ working	☐ reading	☐ meditating
☐ exercising	☐ doing a project	☐ praying
☐ shopping	☐ practicing	☐ with nature
☐ gardening	☐ organizing	☐ being challenged
☐ traveling	☐ thinking	☐ with family + friends
☐ playing	☐ planning	☐ relaxing

More thoughts...etc.....

S M T W T F S _______________ 20___ ___

AM
PM

☐ Sunny   ☐ partly cloudy   ☐ cloudy   ☐ rain   ☐ Snow

-10   zero   10's   20's   30's   40's   50's   60's   70's   80's   90's   100's
☐   ☐   ☐   ☐   ☐   ☐   ☐   ☐   ☐   ☐   ☐   ☐

I FEEL
Happy
Confident
Excited
Enthusiastic
Powerful
Fantastic
Lucky
Hopeful
Content
Focused
Good
Grateful
Confused
Sad
Ashamed
Lonely
Frustrated
Angry
Hurt
Jealous
Exhausted
Overwhelmed
Tired
Scared

I Spent most of today with
____
____
____
____
____

What I like the most today
____
____
____
____

What I like the least today
____
____
____

TODAY'S CHOICES

Physically	Mentally	Spiritually
☐ working	☐ reading	☐ meditating
☐ exercising	☐ doing a project	☐ praying
☐ shopping	☐ practicing	☐ with nature
☐ gardening	☐ organizing	☐ being challenged
☐ traveling	☐ thinking	☐ with family + friends
☐ playing	☐ planning	☐ relaxing

More thoughts...etc.....

SMTWTFS _______________________ 20____ ____ AM / PM

☐ Sunny ☐ partly cloudy ☐ cloudy ☐ rain ☐ Snow

-10 zero 10's 20's 30's 40's 50's 60's 70's 80's 90's 100's
☐   ☐   ☐   ☐   ☐   ☐   ☐   ☐   ☐   ☐   ☐   ☐

I FEEL

Happy
Confident
Excited
Enthusiastic
Powerful
Fantastic
Lucky
Hopeful
Content
Focused
Good
Grateful
Confused
Sad
Ashamed
Lonely
Frustrated
Angry
Hurt
Jealous
Exhausted
Overwhelmed
Tired
Scared

I Spent most of today with

____
____
____
____
____

What I like the most today

____
____
____
____

What I like the least today

____
____
____
____

TODAY'S CHOICES

Physically	Mentally	Spiritually
☐ working	☐ reading	☐ meditating
☐ exercising	☐ doing a project	☐ praying
☐ shopping	☐ practicing	☐ with nature
☐ gardening	☐ organizing	☐ being challenged
☐ traveling	☐ thinking	☐ with family + friends
☐ playing	☐ planning	☐ relaxing

More thoughts...etc.....

SMTWTFS _________________ 20___ ___ AM PM

☐ Sunny   ☐ partly cloudy   ☐ cloudy   ☐ rain   ☐ Snow

-10 zero 10's 20's 30's 40's 50's 60's 70's 80's 90's 100's
☐   ☐   ☐   ☐   ☐   ☐   ☐   ☐   ☐   ☐   ☐   ☐

I FEEL
Happy
Confident
Excited
Enthusiastic
Powerful
Fantastic
Lucky
Hopeful
Content
Focused
Good
Grateful
Confused
Sad
Ashamed
Lonely
Frustrated
Angry
Hurt
Jealous
Exhausted
Overwhelmed
Tired
Scared

I Spent most of today with

____

____

____

____

What I like the most today

____

____

____

____

What I like the least today

____

____

____

TODAY'S CHOICES

Physically	Mentally	Spiritually
☐ working	☐ reading	☐ meditating
☐ exercising	☐ doing a project	☐ praying
☐ shopping	☐ practicing	☐ with nature
☐ gardening	☐ organizing	☐ being challenged
☐ traveling	☐ thinking	☐ with family + friends
☐ playing	☐ planning	☐ relaxing

More thoughts...etc.....

SMTWTFS _________________ 20 ___ ___   AM / PM

☐ Sunny   ☐ partly cloudy   ☐ cloudy   ☐ rain   ☐ Snow

-10   zero   10's   20's   30's   40's   50's   60's   70's   80's   90's   100's
☐   ☐   ☐   ☐   ☐   ☐   ☐   ☐   ☐   ☐   ☐   ☐

I FEEL
Happy
Confident
Excited
Enthusiastic
Powerful
Fantastic
Lucky
Hopeful
Content
Focused
Good
Grateful
Confused
Sad
Ashamed
Lonely
Frustrated
Angry
Hurt
Jealous
Exhausted
Overwhelmed
Tired
Scared

I Spent most of today with

____
____
____
____
____

What I like the most today

____
____
____
____

What I like the least today

____
____
____

TODAY'S CHOICES

Physically	Mentally	Spiritually
☐ working	☐ reading	☐ meditating
☐ exercising	☐ doing a project	☐ praying
☐ shopping	☐ practicing	☐ with nature
☐ gardening	☐ organizing	☐ being challenged
☐ traveling	☐ thinking	☐ with family + friends
☐ playing	☐ planning	☐ relaxing

____

____

____

More thoughts...etc.....

____

____

____

____

SMTWTFS __________________ 20__ __ AM PM

☐ Sunny   ☐ partly cloudy   ☐ cloudy   ☐ rain   ☐ Snow

-10 zero 10's 20's 30's 40's 50's 60's 70's 80's 90's 100's
☐   ☐   ☐   ☐   ☐   ☐   ☐   ☐   ☐   ☐   ☐   ☐

I FEEL
Happy
Confident
Excited
Enthusiastic
Powerful
Fantastic
Lucky
Hopeful
Content
Focused
Good
Grateful
Confused
Sad
Ashamed
Lonely
Frustrated
Angry
Hurt
Jealous
Exhausted
Overwhelmed
Tired
Scared

I Spent most of today with
____
____
____
____
____

What I like the most today
____
____
____
____

What I like the least today
____
____
____
____

TODAY'S CHOICES

Physically	Mentally	Spiritually
☐ working	☐ reading	☐ meditating
☐ exercising	☐ doing a project	☐ praying
☐ shopping	☐ practicing	☐ with nature
☐ gardening	☐ organizing	☐ being challenged
☐ traveling	☐ thinking	☐ with family + friends
☐ playing	☐ planning	☐ relaxing

More thoughts...etc.....

SMTWTFS _________________ 20___ ___ AM / PM

□ Sunny   □ partly cloudy   □ cloudy   □ rain   □ Snow

-10 zero 10's 20's 30's 40's 50's 60's 70's 80's 90's 100's
□   □   □   □   □   □   □   □   □   □   □   □

I FEEL

Happy
Confident
Excited
Enthusiastic
Powerful
Fantastic
Lucky
Hopeful
Content
Focused
Good
Grateful
Confused
Sad
Ashamed
Lonely
Frustrated
Angry
Hurt
Jealous
Exhausted
Overwhelmed
Tired
Scared

I Spent most of today with

____
____
____
____

What I like the most today

____
____
____
____

What I like the least today

____
____
____

TODAY'S CHOICES

Physically	Mentally	Spiritually
☐ working	☐ reading	☐ meditating
☐ exercising	☐ doing a project	☐ praying
☐ shopping	☐ practicing	☐ with nature
☐ gardening	☐ organizing	☐ being challenged
☐ traveling	☐ thinking	☐ with family + friends
☐ playing	☐ planning	☐ relaxing

More thoughts...etc.....

SMTWTFS _______________ 20___ ___ AM / PM

☐ Sunny ☐ partly cloudy ☐ cloudy ☐ rain ☐ Snow

-10 zero 10's 20's 30's 40's 50's 60's 70's 80's 90's 100's
☐   ☐   ☐   ☐   ☐   ☐   ☐   ☐   ☐   ☐   ☐   ☐

I FEEL
Happy
Confident
Excited
Enthusiastic
Powerful
Fantastic
Lucky
Hopeful
Content
Focused
Good
Grateful
Confused
Sad
Ashamed
Lonely
Frustrated
Angry
Hurt
Jealous
Exhausted
Overwhelmed
Tired
Scared

I Spent most of today with

____
____
____
____
____

What I like the most today

____
____
____
____

What I like the least today

____
____
____

TODAY'S CHOICES

Physically	Mentally	Spiritually
☐ working	☐ reading	☐ meditating
☐ exercising	☐ doing a project	☐ praying
☐ shopping	☐ practicing	☐ with nature
☐ gardening	☐ organizing	☐ being challenged
☐ traveling	☐ thinking	☐ with family + friends
☐ playing	☐ planning	☐ relaxing

More thoughts...etc.....

SMTWTFS _________________ 20___ ___ AM / PM

☐ Sunny ☐ partly cloudy ☐ cloudy ☐ rain ☐ Snow

-10 zero 10's 20's 30's 40's 50's 60's 70's 80's 90's 100's
☐   ☐   ☐   ☐   ☐   ☐   ☐   ☐   ☐   ☐   ☐   ☐

I FEEL
- Happy
- Confident
- Excited
- Enthusiastic
- Powerful
- Fantastic
- Lucky
- Hopeful
- Content
- Focused
- Good
- Grateful
- Confused
- Sad
- Ashamed
- Lonely
- Frustrated
- Angry
- Hurt
- Jealous
- Exhausted
- Overwhelmed
- Tired
- Scared

I Spent most of today with

____
____
____
____
____

What I like the most today

____
____
____
____

What I like the least today

____
____
____

TODAY'S CHOICES

Physically	Mentally	Spiritually
☐ working	☐ reading	☐ meditating
☐ exercising	☐ doing a project	☐ praying
☐ shopping	☐ practicing	☐ with nature
☐ gardening	☐ organizing	☐ being challenged
☐ traveling	☐ thinking	☐ with family + friends
☐ playing	☐ planning	☐ relaxing

More thoughts...etc.....

SMTWTFS _________________ 20___ ___ AM / PM

☐ Sunny   ☐ partly cloudy   ☐ cloudy   ☐ rain   ☐ Snow

-10 zero 10's 20's 30's 40's 50's 60's 70's 80's 90's 100's
☐   ☐   ☐   ☐   ☐   ☐   ☐   ☐   ☐   ☐   ☐   ☐

I FEEL

Happy
Confident
Excited
Enthusiastic
Powerful
Fantastic
Lucky
Hopeful
Content
Focused
Good
Grateful
Confused
Sad
Ashamed
Lonely
Frustrated
Angry
Hurt
Jealous
Exhausted
Overwhelmed
Tired
Scared

I Spent most of today with

____

____

____

____

____

What I like the most today

____

____

____

____

What I like the least today

____

____

____

TODAY'S CHOICES

Physically	Mentally	Spiritually
☐ working	☐ reading	☐ meditating
☐ exercising	☐ doing a project	☐ praying
☐ shopping	☐ practicing	☐ with nature
☐ gardening	☐ organizing	☐ being challenged
☐ traveling	☐ thinking	☐ with family + friends
☐ playing	☐ planning	☐ relaxing

More thoughts...etc.....

SMTWTFS _________________ 20 ___ ___ AM / PM

☐ Sunny ☐ partly cloudy ☐ cloudy ☐ rain ☐ Snow

-10 zero 10's 20's 30's 40's 50's 60's 70's 80's 90's 100's
☐   ☐   ☐   ☐   ☐   ☐   ☐   ☐   ☐   ☐   ☐   ☐

I FEEL

Happy
Confident
Excited
Enthusiastic
Powerful
Fantastic
Lucky
Hopeful
Content
Focused
Good
Grateful
Confused
Sad
Ashamed
Lonely
Frustrated
Angry
Hurt
Jealous
Exhausted
Overwhelmed
Tired
Scared

I Spent most of today with

____
____
____
____
____

What I like the most today

____
____
____
____

What I like the least today

____
____
____
____

TODAY'S CHOICES

Physically	Mentally	Spiritually
☐ working	☐ reading	☐ meditating
☐ exercising	☐ doing a project	☐ praying
☐ shopping	☐ practicing	☐ with nature
☐ gardening	☐ organizing	☐ being challenged
☐ traveling	☐ thinking	☐ with family + friends
☐ playing	☐ planning	☐ relaxing

More thoughts...etc.....

SMTWTFS ________________ 20 ___ ___ AM PM

☐ Sunny ☐ partly cloudy ☐ cloudy ☐ rain ☐ Snow

-10 zero 10's 20's 30's 40's 50's 60's 70's 80's 90's 100's
☐   ☐   ☐   ☐   ☐   ☐   ☐   ☐   ☐   ☐   ☐   ☐

I FEEL
Happy
Confident
Excited
Enthusiastic
Powerful
Fantastic
Lucky
Hopeful
Content
Focused
Good
Grateful
Confused
Sad
Ashamed
Lonely
Frustrated
Angry
Hurt
Jealous
Exhausted
Overwhelmed
Tired
Scared

I Spent most of today with

____
____
____
____
____

What I like the most today

____
____
____
____

What I like the least today

____
____
____

TODAY'S CHOICES

Physically	Mentally	Spiritually
☐ working	☐ reading	☐ meditating
☐ exercising	☐ doing a project	☐ praying
☐ shopping	☐ practicing	☐ with nature
☐ gardening	☐ organizing	☐ being challenged
☐ traveling	☐ thinking	☐ with family + friends
☐ playing	☐ planning	☐ relaxing

More thoughts...etc.....

SMTWTFS ___________ 20___ ___
AM
PM

☐ Sunny ☐ partly cloudy ☐ cloudy ☐ rain ☐ Snow

-10 zero 10's 20's 30's 40's 50's 60's 70's 80's 90's 100's
☐ ☐ ☐ ☐ ☐ ☐ ☐ ☐ ☐ ☐ ☐ ☐

I FEEL

- Happy
- Confident
- Excited
- Enthusiastic
- Powerful
- Fantastic
- Lucky
- Hopeful
- Content
- Focused
- Good
- Grateful
- Confused
- Sad
- Ashamed
- Lonely
- Frustrated
- Angry
- Hurt
- Jealous
- Exhausted
- Overwhelmed
- Tired
- Scared

I Spent most of today with

____
____
____
____
____

What I like the most today

____
____
____
____

What I like the least today

____
____
____

TODAY'S CHOICES

Physically	Mentally	Spiritually
☐ working	☐ reading	☐ meditating
☐ exercising	☐ doing a project	☐ praying
☐ shopping	☐ practicing	☐ with nature
☐ gardening	☐ organizing	☐ being challenged
☐ traveling	☐ thinking	☐ with family + friends
☐ playing	☐ planning	☐ relaxing

More thoughts...etc.....

SMTWTFS __________________ 20 __ __   AM / PM

□ Sunny   □ partly cloudy   □ cloudy   □ rain   □ Snow

-10 zero 10's 20's 30's 40's 50's 60's 70's 80's 90's 100's
□   □   □   □   □   □   □   □   □   □   □   □

I FEEL

- Happy
- Confident
- Excited
- Enthusiastic
- Powerful
- Fantastic
- Lucky
- Hopeful
- Content
- Focused
- Good
- Grateful
- Confused
- Sad
- Ashamed
- Lonely
- Frustrated
- Angry
- Hurt
- Jealous
- Exhausted
- Overwhelmed
- Tired
- Scared

I Spent most of today with
____
____
____
____
____

What I like the most today
____
____
____
____

What I like the least today
____
____
____

TODAY'S CHOICES

Physically	Mentally	Spiritually
☐ working	☐ reading	☐ meditating
☐ exercising	☐ doing a project	☐ praying
☐ shopping	☐ practicing	☐ with nature
☐ gardening	☐ organizing	☐ being challenged
☐ traveling	☐ thinking	☐ with family + friends
☐ playing	☐ planning	☐ relaxing

More thoughts...etc.....

SMTWTFS _______________ 20__ __ AM PM

☐ Sunny ☐ partly cloudy ☐ cloudy ☐ rain ☐ Snow

-10 zero 10's 20's 30's 40's 50's 60's 70's 80's 90's 100's
☐   ☐   ☐   ☐   ☐   ☐   ☐   ☐   ☐   ☐   ☐   ☐

I FEEL
- Happy
- Confident
- Excited
- Enthusiastic
- Powerful
- Fantastic
- Lucky
- Hopeful
- Content
- Focused
- Good
- Grateful
- Confused
- Sad
- Ashamed
- Lonely
- Frustrated
- Angry
- Hurt
- Jealous
- Exhausted
- Overwhelmed
- Tired
- Scared

I Spent most of today with

____

____

____

____

____

What I like the most today

____

____

____

____

What I like the least today

____

____

____

TODAY'S CHOICES

Physically	Mentally	Spiritually
☐ working	☐ reading	☐ meditating
☐ exercising	☐ doing a project	☐ praying
☐ shopping	☐ practicing	☐ with nature
☐ gardening	☐ organizing	☐ being challenged
☐ traveling	☐ thinking	☐ with family + friends
☐ playing	☐ planning	☐ relaxing

More thoughts...etc.....

SMTWTFS _______________ 20 ___ ___ AM / PM

☐ Sunny ☐ partly cloudy ☐ cloudy ☐ rain ☐ Snow

-10 zero 10's 20's 30's 40's 50's 60's 70's 80's 90's 100's
☐   ☐   ☐   ☐   ☐   ☐   ☐   ☐   ☐   ☐   ☐   ☐

I FEEL

Happy
Confident
Excited
Enthusiastic
Powerful
Fantastic
Lucky
Hopeful
Content
Focused
Good
Grateful
Confused
Sad
Ashamed
Lonely
Frustrated
Angry
Hurt
Jealous
Exhausted
Overwhelmed
Tired
Scared

I Spent most of today with

____
____
____
____
____

What I like the most today

____
____
____
____

What I like the least today

____
____
____
____

TODAY'S CHOICES

Physically	Mentally	Spiritually
☐ working	☐ reading	☐ meditating
☐ exercising	☐ doing a project	☐ praying
☐ shopping	☐ practicing	☐ with nature
☐ gardening	☐ organizing	☐ being challenged
☐ traveling	☐ thinking	☐ with family + friends
☐ playing	☐ planning	☐ relaxing

More thoughts...etc.....

SMTWTFS _________________ 20___ ___ AM/PM

☐ Sunny ☐ partly cloudy ☐ cloudy ☐ rain ☐ Snow

-10 zero 10's 20's 30's 40's 50's 60's 70's 80's 90's 100's
☐ ☐ ☐ ☐ ☐ ☐ ☐ ☐ ☐ ☐ ☐ ☐

I FEEL

- Happy
- Confident
- Excited
- Enthusiastic
- Powerful
- Fantastic
- Lucky
- Hopeful
- Content
- Focused
- Good
- Grateful
- Confused
- Sad
- Ashamed
- Lonely
- Frustrated
- Angry
- Hurt
- Jealous
- Exhausted
- Overwhelmed
- Tired
- Scared

I Spent most of today with

____

____

____

____

____

What I like the most today

____

____

____

____

What I like the least today

____

____

____

TODAY'S CHOICES

Physically	Mentally	Spiritually
☐ working	☐ reading	☐ meditating
☐ exercising	☐ doing a project	☐ praying
☐ shopping	☐ practicing	☐ with nature
☐ gardening	☐ organizing	☐ being challenged
☐ traveling	☐ thinking	☐ with family + friends
☐ playing	☐ planning	☐ relaxing

More thoughts...etc.....

SMTWTFS __________________ 20___ ___ AM / PM

☐ Sunny ☐ partly cloudy ☐ cloudy ☐ rain ☐ Snow

-10 zero 10's 20's 30's 40's 50's 60's 70's 80's 90's 100's
☐ ☐ ☐ ☐ ☐ ☐ ☐ ☐ ☐ ☐ ☐ ☐

I FEEL
Happy
Confident
Excited
Enthusiastic
Powerful
Fantastic
Lucky
Hopeful
Content
Focused
Good
Grateful
Confused
Sad
Ashamed
Lonely
Frustrated
Angry
Hurt
Jealous
Exhausted
Overwhelmed
Tired
Scared

I Spent most of today with
____
____
____
____
____

What I like the most today
____
____
____
____

What I like the least today
____
____
____
____

TODAY'S CHOICES

Physically	Mentally	Spiritually
☐ working	☐ reading	☐ meditating
☐ exercising	☐ doing a project	☐ praying
☐ shopping	☐ practicing	☐ with nature
☐ gardening	☐ organizing	☐ being challenged
☐ traveling	☐ thinking	☐ with family + friends
☐ playing	☐ planning	☐ relaxing

_______________   _______________   _______________

_______________   _______________   _______________

_______________   _______________   _______________

More thoughts...etc.....

____

____

____

____

SMTWTFS __________________ 20___ ___

AM
PM

☐ Sunny ☐ partly cloudy ☐ cloudy ☐ rain ☐ Snow

-10 zero 10's 20's 30's 40's 50's 60's 70's 80's 90's 100's
☐   ☐   ☐   ☐   ☐   ☐   ☐   ☐   ☐   ☐   ☐   ☐

I FEEL
Happy
Confident
Excited
Enthusiastic
Powerful
Fantastic
Lucky
Hopeful
Content
Focused
Good
Grateful
Confused
Sad
Ashamed
Lonely
Frustrated
Angry
Hurt
Jealous
Exhausted
Overwhelmed
Tired
Scared

I Spent most of today with

____
____
____
____
____

What I like the most today

____
____
____
____

What I like the least today

____
____
____
____

TODAY'S CHOICES

Physically	Mentally	Spiritually
☐ working	☐ reading	☐ meditating
☐ exercising	☐ doing a project	☐ praying
☐ shopping	☐ practicing	☐ with nature
☐ gardening	☐ organizing	☐ being challenged
☐ traveling	☐ thinking	☐ with family + friends
☐ playing	☐ planning	☐ relaxing

More thoughts...etc.....

SMTWTFS _______________________ 20___ ___ AM / PM

☐ Sunny   ☐ partly cloudy   ☐ cloudy   ☐ rain   ☐ Snow

-10   zero   10's   20's   30's   40's   50's   60's   70's   80's   90's   100's
☐   ☐   ☐   ☐   ☐   ☐   ☐   ☐   ☐   ☐   ☐   ☐

I FEEL

Happy
Confident
Excited
Enthusiastic
Powerful
Fantastic
Lucky
Hopeful
Content
Focused
Good
Grateful
Confused
Sad
Ashamed
Lonely
Frustrated
Angry
Hurt
Jealous
Exhausted
Overwhelmed
Tired
Scared

I Spent most of today with

____
____
____
____
____

What I like the most today

____
____
____
____

What I like the least today

____
____
____

TODAY'S CHOICES

Physically	Mentally	Spiritually
☐ working	☐ reading	☐ meditating
☐ exercising	☐ doing a project	☐ praying
☐ shopping	☐ practicing	☐ with nature
☐ gardening	☐ organizing	☐ being challenged
☐ traveling	☐ thinking	☐ with family + friends
☐ playing	☐ planning	☐ relaxing

_______________   _______________   _______________

_______________   _______________   _______________

_______________   _______________   _______________

More thoughts...etc.....

____

____

____

____

SMTWTFS _________________________ 20___ ___ AM / PM

☐ Sunny   ☐ partly cloudy   ☐ cloudy   ☐ rain   ☐ Snow

-10 zero 10's 20's 30's 40's 50's 60's 70's 80's 90's 100's
☐   ☐   ☐   ☐   ☐   ☐   ☐   ☐   ☐   ☐   ☐   ☐

I FEEL
- Happy
- Confident
- Excited
- Enthusiastic
- Powerful
- Fantastic
- Lucky
- Hopeful
- Content
- Focused
- Good
- Grateful
- Confused
- Sad
- Ashamed
- Lonely
- Frustrated
- Angry
- Hurt
- Jealous
- Exhausted
- Overwhelmed
- Tired
- Scared

I Spent most of today with

____

____

____

____

____

What I like the most today

____

____

____

____

What I like the least today

____

____

____

____

TODAY'S CHOICES

Physically	Mentally	Spiritually
☐ working	☐ reading	☐ meditating
☐ exercising	☐ doing a project	☐ praying
☐ shopping	☐ practicing	☐ with nature
☐ gardening	☐ organizing	☐ being challenged
☐ traveling	☐ thinking	☐ with family + friends
☐ playing	☐ planning	☐ relaxing

More thoughts...etc.....

SMTWTFS _________________ 20__ __ AM / PM

☐ Sunny   ☐ partly cloudy   ☐ cloudy   ☐ rain   ☐ Snow

-10 zero 10's 20's 30's 40's 50's 60's 70's 80's 90's 100's
☐   ☐   ☐   ☐   ☐   ☐   ☐   ☐   ☐   ☐   ☐   ☐

I FEEL

- Happy
- Confident
- Excited
- Enthusiastic
- Powerful
- Fantastic
- Lucky
- Hopeful
- Content
- Focused
- Good
- Grateful
- Confused
- Sad
- Ashamed
- Lonely
- Frustrated
- Angry
- Hurt
- Jealous
- Exhausted
- Overwhelmed
- Tired
- Scared

I Spent most of today with

____

____

____

____

____

What I like the most today

____

____

____

____

What I like the least today

____

____

____

TODAY'S CHOICES

Physically	Mentally	Spiritually
☐ working	☐ reading	☐ meditating
☐ exercising	☐ doing a project	☐ praying
☐ shopping	☐ practicing	☐ with nature
☐ gardening	☐ organizing	☐ being challenged
☐ traveling	☐ thinking	☐ with family + friends
☐ playing	☐ planning	☐ relaxing

More thoughts...etc.....

SMTWTFS _____________ 20___ ___   AM / PM

☐ Sunny   ☐ partly cloudy   ☐ cloudy   ☐ rain   ☐ Snow

-10   zero   10's   20's   30's   40's   50's   60's   70's   80's   90's   100's
☐   ☐   ☐   ☐   ☐   ☐   ☐   ☐   ☐   ☐   ☐   ☐

I FEEL

- Happy
- Confident
- Excited
- Enthusiastic
- Powerful
- Fantastic
- Lucky
- Hopeful
- Content
- Focused
- Good
- Grateful
- Confused
- Sad
- Ashamed
- Lonely
- Frustrated
- Angry
- Hurt
- Jealous
- Exhausted
- Overwhelmed
- Tired
- Scared

I Spent most of today with

____
____
____
____
____

What I like the most today

____
____
____
____

What I like the least today

____
____
____

TODAY'S CHOICES

Physically	Mentally	Spiritually
☐ working	☐ reading	☐ meditating
☐ exercising	☐ doing a project	☐ praying
☐ shopping	☐ practicing	☐ with nature
☐ gardening	☐ organizing	☐ being challenged
☐ traveling	☐ thinking	☐ with family + friends
☐ playing	☐ planning	☐ relaxing

More thoughts...etc.....

SMTWTFS ________________ 20___ ___ AM PM

☐ Sunny   ☐ partly cloudy   ☐ cloudy   ☐ rain   ☐ Snow

-10   zero   10's   20's   30's   40's   50's   60's   70's   80's   90's   100's
☐   ☐   ☐   ☐   ☐   ☐   ☐   ☐   ☐   ☐   ☐   ☐

I FEEL
Happy
Confident
Excited
Enthusiastic
Powerful
Fantastic
Lucky
Hopeful
Content
Focused
Good
Grateful
Confused
Sad
Ashamed
Lonely
Frustrated
Angry
Hurt
Jealous
Exhausted
Overwhelmed
Tired
Scared

I Spent most of today with

____

____

____

____

____

What I like the most today

____

____

____

____

What I like the least today

____

____

____

TODAY'S CHOICES

Physically	Mentally	Spiritually
☐ working	☐ reading	☐ meditating
☐ exercising	☐ doing a project	☐ praying
☐ shopping	☐ practicing	☐ with nature
☐ gardening	☐ organizing	☐ being challenged
☐ traveling	☐ thinking	☐ with family + friends
☐ playing	☐ planning	☐ relaxing

More thoughts...etc.....

SMTWTFS ____________ 20__ __ AM PM

☐ Sunny ☐ partly cloudy ☐ cloudy ☐ rain ☐ Snow

-10 zero 10's 20's 30's 40's 50's 60's 70's 80's 90's 100's
☐ ☐ ☐ ☐ ☐ ☐ ☐ ☐ ☐ ☐ ☐ ☐

I FEEL
Happy
Confident
Excited
Enthusiastic
Powerful
Fantastic
Lucky
Hopeful
Content
Focused
Good
Grateful
Confused
Sad
Ashamed
Lonely
Frustrated
Angry
Hurt
Jealous
Exhausted
Overwhelmed
Tired
Scared

I Spent most of today with

____

____

____

____

____

What I like the most today

____

____

____

____

What I like the least today

____

____

____

TODAY'S CHOICES

Physically	Mentally	Spiritually
☐ working	☐ reading	☐ meditating
☐ exercising	☐ doing a project	☐ praying
☐ shopping	☐ practicing	☐ with nature
☐ gardening	☐ organizing	☐ being challenged
☐ traveling	☐ thinking	☐ with family + friends
☐ playing	☐ planning	☐ relaxing

More thoughts...etc.....

SMTWTFS _________________ 20 __ __ AM / PM

☐ Sunny ☐ partly cloudy ☐ cloudy ☐ rain ☐ Snow

-10 zero 10's 20's 30's 40's 50's 60's 70's 80's 90's 100's
☐   ☐   ☐   ☐   ☐   ☐   ☐   ☐   ☐   ☐   ☐   ☐

I FEEL

I FEEL
Happy
Confident
Excited
Enthusiastic
Powerful
Fantastic
Lucky
Hopeful
Content
Focused
Good
Grateful
Confused
Sad
Ashamed
Lonely
Frustrated
Angry
Hurt
Jealous
Exhausted
Overwhelmed
Tired
Scared

I Spent most of today with
____
____
____
____
____

What I like the most today
____
____
____
____

What I like the least today
____
____
____
____

TODAY'S CHOICES

Physically	Mentally	Spiritually
☐ working	☐ reading	☐ meditating
☐ exercising	☐ doing a project	☐ praying
☐ shopping	☐ practicing	☐ with nature
☐ gardening	☐ organizing	☐ being challenged
☐ traveling	☐ thinking	☐ with family + friends
☐ playing	☐ planning	☐ relaxing

More thoughts...etc.....

SMTWTFS ______________________ 20___ ___

AM
PM

☐ Sunny   ☐ partly cloudy   ☐ cloudy   ☐ rain   ☐ Snow

-10   zero   10's   20's   30's   40's   50's   60's   70's   80's   90's   100's
☐   ☐   ☐   ☐   ☐   ☐   ☐   ☐   ☐   ☐   ☐   ☐

I FEEL
Happy
Confident
Excited
Enthusiastic
Powerful
Fantastic
Lucky
Hopeful
Content
Focused
Good
Grateful
Confused
Sad
Ashamed
Lonely
Frustrated
Angry
Hurt
Jealous
Exhausted
Overwhelmed
Tired
Scared

I Spent most of today with

____
____
____
____
____

What I like the most today

____
____
____
____

What I like the least today

____
____
____

TODAY'S CHOICES

Physically	Mentally	Spiritually
☐ working	☐ reading	☐ meditating
☐ exercising	☐ doing a project	☐ praying
☐ shopping	☐ practicing	☐ with nature
☐ gardening	☐ organizing	☐ being challenged
☐ traveling	☐ thinking	☐ with family + friends
☐ playing	☐ planning	☐ relaxing

More thoughts...etc.....

SMTWTFS _________________ 20___ ___ AM PM

☐ Sunny ☐ partly cloudy ☐ cloudy ☐ rain ☐ Snow

-10 zero 10's 20's 30's 40's 50's 60's 70's 80's 90's 100's
☐ ☐ ☐ ☐ ☐ ☐ ☐ ☐ ☐ ☐ ☐ ☐

I FEEL
Happy
Confident
Excited
Enthusiastic
Powerful
Fantastic
Lucky
Hopeful
Content
Focused
Good
Grateful
Confused
Sad
Ashamed
Lonely
Frustrated
Angry
Hurt
Jealous
Exhausted
Overwhelmed
Tired
Scared

I Spent most of today with

____
____
____
____
____

What I like the most today

____
____
____
____

What I like the least today

____
____
____

TODAY'S CHOICES

Physically	Mentally	Spiritually
☐ working	☐ reading	☐ meditating
☐ exercising	☐ doing a project	☐ praying
☐ shopping	☐ practicing	☐ with nature
☐ gardening	☐ organizing	☐ being challenged
☐ traveling	☐ thinking	☐ with family + friends
☐ playing	☐ planning	☐ relaxing

More thoughts...etc.....

SMTWTFS _________________ 20___ ___ AM / PM

☐ Sunny ☐ partly cloudy ☐ cloudy ☐ rain ☐ Snow

-10 zero 10's 20's 30's 40's 50's 60's 70's 80's 90's 100's
☐   ☐   ☐   ☐   ☐   ☐   ☐   ☐   ☐   ☐   ☐   ☐

I FEEL

Happy
Confident
Excited
Enthusiastic
Powerful
Fantastic
Lucky
Hopeful
Content
Focused
Good
Grateful
Confused
Sad
Ashamed
Lonely
Frustrated
Angry
Hurt
Jealous
Exhausted
Overwhelmed
Tired
Scared

I Spent most of today with

____
____
____
____
____

What I like the most today

____
____
____
____

What I like the least today

____
____
____

TODAY'S CHOICES

Physically	Mentally	Spiritually
☐ working	☐ reading	☐ meditating
☐ exercising	☐ doing a project	☐ praying
☐ shopping	☐ practicing	☐ with nature
☐ gardening	☐ organizing	☐ being challenged
☐ traveling	☐ thinking	☐ with family + friends
☐ playing	☐ planning	☐ relaxing

More thoughts...etc.....

SMTWTFS_______________ 20___ ___ AM / PM

☐ Sunny ☐ partly cloudy ☐ cloudy ☐ rain ☐ Snow

-10 zero 10's 20's 30's 40's 50's 60's 70's 80's 90's 100's
☐   ☐   ☐   ☐   ☐   ☐   ☐   ☐   ☐   ☐   ☐   ☐

I FEEL

- Happy
- Confident
- Excited
- Enthusiastic
- Powerful
- Fantastic
- Lucky
- Hopeful
- Content
- Focused
- Good
- Grateful
- Confused
- Sad
- Ashamed
- Lonely
- Frustrated
- Angry
- Hurt
- Jealous
- Exhausted
- Overwhelmed
- Tired
- Scared

I Spent most of today with

____

____

____

____

____

What I like the most today

____

____

____

____

What I like the least today

____

____

____

____

TODAY'S CHOICES

Physically	Mentally	Spiritually
☐ working	☐ reading	☐ meditating
☐ exercising	☐ doing a project	☐ praying
☐ shopping	☐ practicing	☐ with nature
☐ gardening	☐ organizing	☐ being challenged
☐ traveling	☐ thinking	☐ with family + friends
☐ playing	☐ planning	☐ relaxing

_______________   _______________   _______________

_______________   _______________   _______________

_______________   _______________   _______________

More thoughts...etc.....

____

____

____

____

SMTWTFS _________________ 20___ ___ AM / PM

☐ Sunny ☐ partly cloudy ☐ cloudy ☐ rain ☐ Snow

-10 zero 10's 20's 30's 40's 50's 60's 70's 80's 90's 100's
☐   ☐   ☐   ☐   ☐   ☐   ☐   ☐   ☐   ☐   ☐   ☐

I FEEL
- Happy
- Confident
- Excited
- Enthusiastic
- Powerful
- Fantastic
- Lucky
- Hopeful
- Content
- Focused
- Good
- Grateful
- Confused
- Sad
- Ashamed
- Lonely
- Frustrated
- Angry
- Hurt
- Jealous
- Exhausted
- Overwhelmed
- Tired
- Scared

I Spent most of today with

____

____

____

____

____

What I like the most today

____

____

____

____

What I like the least today

____

____

____

TODAY'S CHOICES

Physically	Mentally	Spiritually
☐ working	☐ reading	☐ meditating
☐ exercising	☐ doing a project	☐ praying
☐ shopping	☐ practicing	☐ with nature
☐ gardening	☐ organizing	☐ being challenged
☐ traveling	☐ thinking	☐ with family + friends
☐ playing	☐ planning	☐ relaxing

More thoughts...etc.....

SMTWTFS _______________ 20___ ___ AM PM

☐ Sunny   ☐ partly cloudy   ☐ cloudy   ☐ rain   ☐ Snow

-10 zero 10's 20's 30's 40's 50's 60's 70's 80's 90's 100's
☐   ☐   ☐   ☐   ☐   ☐   ☐   ☐   ☐   ☐   ☐   ☐

I FEEL
Happy
Confident
Excited
Enthusiastic
Powerful
Fantastic
Lucky
Hopeful
Content
Focused
Good
Grateful
Confused
Sad
Ashamed
Lonely
Frustrated
Angry
Hurt
Jealous
Exhausted
Overwhelmed
Tired
Scared

I Spent most of today with

____
____
____
____
____

What I like the most today

____
____
____
____

What I like the least today

____
____
____

TODAY'S CHOICES

Physically	Mentally	Spiritually
☐ working	☐ reading	☐ meditating
☐ exercising	☐ doing a project	☐ praying
☐ shopping	☐ practicing	☐ with nature
☐ gardening	☐ organizing	☐ being challenged
☐ traveling	☐ thinking	☐ with family + friends
☐ playing	☐ planning	☐ relaxing

More thoughts...etc.....

SMTWTFS _______________ 20 ___ ___ AM PM

☐ Sunny   ☐ partly cloudy   ☐ cloudy   ☐ rain   ☐ Snow

-10   zero   10's   20's   30's   40's   50's   60's   70's   80's   90's   100's
☐   ☐   ☐   ☐   ☐   ☐   ☐   ☐   ☐   ☐   ☐   ☐

I FEEL

Happy
Confident
Excited
Enthusiastic
Powerful
Fantastic
Lucky
Hopeful
Content
Focused
Good
Grateful
Confused
Sad
Ashamed
Lonely
Frustrated
Angry
Hurt
Jealous
Exhausted
Overwhelmed
Tired
Scared

I Spent most of today with

____

____

____

____

What I like the most today

____

____

____

____

What I like the least today

____

____

____

TODAY'S CHOICES

Physically	Mentally	Spiritually
☐ working	☐ reading	☐ meditating
☐ exercising	☐ doing a project	☐ praying
☐ shopping	☐ practicing	☐ with nature
☐ gardening	☐ organizing	☐ being challenged
☐ traveling	☐ thinking	☐ with family + friends
☐ playing	☐ planning	☐ relaxing

More thoughts...etc.....

SMTWTFS _________________ 20___ ___ AM PM

☐ Sunny ☐ partly cloudy ☐ cloudy ☐ rain ☐ Snow

-10 zero 10's 20's 30's 40's 50's 60's 70's 80's 90's 100's
☐   ☐   ☐   ☐   ☐   ☐   ☐   ☐   ☐   ☐   ☐   ☐

I FEEL
Happy
Confident
Excited
Enthusiastic
Powerful
Fantastic
Lucky
Hopeful
Content
Focused
Good
Grateful
Confused
Sad
Ashamed
Lonely
Frustrated
Angry
Hurt
Jealous
Exhausted
Overwhelmed
Tired
Scared

I Spent most of today with

____
____
____
____
____

What I like the most today

____
____
____
____

What I like the least today

____
____
____

TODAY'S CHOICES

Physically	Mentally	Spiritually
☐ working	☐ reading	☐ meditating
☐ exercising	☐ doing a project	☐ praying
☐ shopping	☐ practicing	☐ with nature
☐ gardening	☐ organizing	☐ being challenged
☐ traveling	☐ thinking	☐ with family + friends
☐ playing	☐ planning	☐ relaxing

More thoughts...etc.....

SMTWTFS _________________ 20___ ___ AM PM

☀ ⛅ ☁ 🌧 ❄

☐ Sunny   ☐ partly cloudy   ☐ cloudy   ☐ rain   ☐ Snow

-10   zero   10's   20's   30's   40's   50's   60's   70's   80's   90's   100's
☐   ☐   ☐   ☐   ☐   ☐   ☐   ☐   ☐   ☐   ☐   ☐

I FEEL
Happy
Confident
Excited
Enthusiastic
Powerful
Fantastic
Lucky
Hopeful
Content
Focused
Good
Grateful
Confused
Sad
Ashamed
Lonely
Frustrated
Angry
Hurt
Jealous
Exhausted
Overwhelmed
Tired
Scared

I Spent most of today with

____
____
____
____
____

What I like the most today

____
____
____
____

What I like the least today

____
____
____

TODAY'S CHOICES

Physically	Mentally	Spiritually
☐ working	☐ reading	☐ meditating
☐ exercising	☐ doing a project	☐ praying
☐ shopping	☐ practicing	☐ with nature
☐ gardening	☐ organizing	☐ being challenged
☐ traveling	☐ thinking	☐ with family + friends
☐ playing	☐ planning	☐ relaxing

More thoughts...etc.....

SMTWTFS _________________ 20___ ___

AM
PM

☐ Sunny ☐ partly cloudy ☐ cloudy ☐ rain ☐ Snow

-10 zero 10's 20's 30's 40's 50's 60's 70's 80's 90's 100's
☐   ☐   ☐   ☐   ☐   ☐   ☐   ☐   ☐   ☐   ☐   ☐

I FEEL

Happy
Confident
Excited
Enthusiastic
Powerful
Fantastic
Lucky
Hopeful
Content
Focused
Good
Grateful
Confused
Sad
Ashamed
Lonely
Frustrated
Angry
Hurt
Jealous
Exhausted
Overwhelmed
Tired
Scared

I Spent most of today with

____
____
____
____
____

What I like the most today

____
____
____
____
____

What I like the least today

____
____
____

TODAY'S CHOICES

Physically	Mentally	Spiritually
☐ working	☐ reading	☐ meditating
☐ exercising	☐ doing a project	☐ praying
☐ shopping	☐ practicing	☐ with nature
☐ gardening	☐ organizing	☐ being challenged
☐ traveling	☐ thinking	☐ with family + friends
☐ playing	☐ planning	☐ relaxing

More thoughts...etc.....

SMTWTFS __________________ 20___ ___ AM/PM

☐ Sunny ☐ partly cloudy ☐ cloudy ☐ rain ☐ Snow

-10 zero 10's 20's 30's 40's 50's 60's 70's 80's 90's 100's
☐ ☐ ☐ ☐ ☐ ☐ ☐ ☐ ☐ ☐ ☐ ☐

I FEEL

- Happy
- Confident
- Excited
- Enthusiastic
- Powerful
- Fantastic
- Lucky
- Hopeful
- Content
- Focused
- Good
- Grateful
- Confused
- Sad
- Ashamed
- Lonely
- Frustrated
- Angry
- Hurt
- Jealous
- Exhausted
- Overwhelmed
- Tired
- Scared

I Spent most of today with

____

____

____

____

____

What I like the most today

____

____

____

____

What I like the least today

____

____

____

TODAY'S CHOICES

Physically	Mentally	Spiritually
☐ working	☐ reading	☐ meditating
☐ exercising	☐ doing a project	☐ praying
☐ shopping	☐ practicing	☐ with nature
☐ gardening	☐ organizing	☐ being challenged
☐ traveling	☐ thinking	☐ with family + friends
☐ playing	☐ planning	☐ relaxing

More thoughts...etc.....

SMTWTFS ____________ 20__ __ AM / PM

☐ Sunny ☐ partly cloudy ☐ cloudy ☐ rain ☐ Snow

-10 zero 10's 20's 30's 40's 50's 60's 70's 80's 90's 100's
☐   ☐   ☐   ☐   ☐   ☐   ☐   ☐   ☐   ☐   ☐   ☐

I FEEL
- Happy
- Confident
- Excited
- Enthusiastic
- Powerful
- Fantastic
- Lucky
- Hopeful
- Content
- Focused
- Good
- Grateful
- Confused
- Sad
- Ashamed
- Lonely
- Frustrated
- Angry
- Hurt
- Jealous
- Exhausted
- Overwhelmed
- Tired
- Scared

I Spent most of today with

____

____

____

____

____

What I like the most today

____

____

____

____

What I like the least today

____

____

____

TODAY'S CHOICES

Physically	Mentally	Spiritually
☐ working	☐ reading	☐ meditating
☐ exercising	☐ doing a project	☐ praying
☐ shopping	☐ practicing	☐ with nature
☐ gardening	☐ organizing	☐ being challenged
☐ traveling	☐ thinking	☐ with family + friends
☐ playing	☐ planning	☐ relaxing

More thoughts...etc.....

SMTWTFS _________________ 20___ ___ AM / PM

☐ Sunny ☐ partly cloudy ☐ cloudy ☐ rain ☐ Snow

-10 zero 10's 20's 30's 40's 50's 60's 70's 80's 90's 100's
☐   ☐   ☐   ☐   ☐   ☐   ☐   ☐   ☐   ☐   ☐   ☐

I FEEL

Happy
Confident
Excited
Enthusiastic
Powerful
Fantastic
Lucky
Hopeful
Content
Focused
Good
Grateful
Confused
Sad
Ashamed
Lonely
Frustrated
Angry
Hurt
Jealous
Exhausted
Overwhelmed
Tired
Scared

I Spent most of today with

____
____
____
____
____

What I like the most today

____
____
____
____

What I like the least today

____
____
____
____

TODAY'S CHOICES

Physically	Mentally	Spiritually
☐ working	☐ reading	☐ meditating
☐ exercising	☐ doing a project	☐ praying
☐ shopping	☐ practicing	☐ with nature
☐ gardening	☐ organizing	☐ being challenged
☐ traveling	☐ thinking	☐ with family + friends
☐ playing	☐ planning	☐ relaxing

More thoughts...etc.....

SMTWTFS _______________ 20___ ___ AM / PM

☐ Sunny ☐ partly cloudy ☐ cloudy ☐ rain ☐ Snow

-10 zero 10's 20's 30's 40's 50's 60's 70's 80's 90's 100's
☐   ☐   ☐   ☐   ☐   ☐   ☐   ☐   ☐   ☐   ☐   ☐

I FEEL

Happy
Confident
Excited
Enthusiastic
Powerful
Fantastic
Lucky
Hopeful
Content
Focused
Good
Grateful
Confused
Sad
Ashamed
Lonely
Frustrated
Angry
Hurt
Jealous
Exhausted
Overwhelmed
Tired
Scared

I Spent most of today with

____
____
____
____
____

What I like the most today

____
____
____
____

What I like the least today

____
____
____

TODAY'S CHOICES

Physically	Mentally	Spiritually
☐ working	☐ reading	☐ meditating
☐ exercising	☐ doing a project	☐ praying
☐ shopping	☐ practicing	☐ with nature
☐ gardening	☐ organizing	☐ being challenged
☐ traveling	☐ thinking	☐ with family + friends
☐ playing	☐ planning	☐ relaxing

More thoughts...etc.....

SMTWTFS _________________________ 20___ ___ AM / PM

☐ Sunny   ☐ partly cloudy   ☐ cloudy   ☐ rain   ☐ Snow

-10 zero 10's 20's 30's 40's 50's 60's 70's 80's 90's 100's
☐   ☐   ☐   ☐   ☐   ☐   ☐   ☐   ☐   ☐   ☐   ☐

I FEEL

- Happy
- Confident
- Excited
- Enthusiastic
- Powerful
- Fantastic
- Lucky
- Hopeful
- Content
- Focused
- Good
- Grateful
- Confused
- Sad
- Ashamed
- Lonely
- Frustrated
- Angry
- Hurt
- Jealous
- Exhausted
- Overwhelmed
- Tired
- Scared

I Spent most of today with

____
____
____
____
____

What I like the most today

____
____
____
____

What I like the least today

____
____
____
____

TODAY'S CHOICES

Physically	Mentally	Spiritually
☐ working	☐ reading	☐ meditating
☐ exercising	☐ doing a project	☐ praying
☐ shopping	☐ practicing	☐ with nature
☐ gardening	☐ organizing	☐ being challenged
☐ traveling	☐ thinking	☐ with family + friends
☐ playing	☐ planning	☐ relaxing

_______________ _______________ _______________

_______________ _______________ _______________

_______________ _______________ _______________

More thoughts...etc.....

____

____

____

____

SMTWTFS _________________________ 20___ ___ AM / PM

☐ Sunny   ☐ partly cloudy   ☐ cloudy   ☐ rain   ☐ Snow

-10 zero 10's 20's 30's 40's 50's 60's 70's 80's 90's 100's
☐   ☐   ☐   ☐   ☐   ☐   ☐   ☐   ☐   ☐   ☐   ☐

I FEEL
Happy
Confident
Excited
Enthusiastic
Powerful
Fantastic
Lucky
Hopeful
Content
Focused
Good
Grateful
Confused
Sad
Ashamed
Lonely
Frustrated
Angry
Hurt
Jealous
Exhausted
Overwhelmed
Tired
Scared

I Spent most of today with
____
____
____
____
____

What I like the most today
____
____
____
____

What I like the least today
____
____
____
____

TODAY'S CHOICES

Physically	Mentally	Spiritually
☐ working	☐ reading	☐ meditating
☐ exercising	☐ doing a project	☐ praying
☐ shopping	☐ practicing	☐ with nature
☐ gardening	☐ organizing	☐ being challenged
☐ traveling	☐ thinking	☐ with family + friends
☐ playing	☐ planning	☐ relaxing

More thoughts...etc.....

SMTWTFS _________________ 20___ ___
AM
PM

☐ Sunny ☐ partly cloudy ☐ cloudy ☐ rain ☐ Snow

-10 zero 10's 20's 30's 40's 50's 60's 70's 80's 90's 100's
☐ ☐ ☐ ☐ ☐ ☐ ☐ ☐ ☐ ☐ ☐ ☐

I FEEL

Happy
Confident
Excited
Enthusiastic
Powerful
Fantastic
Lucky
Hopeful
Content
Focused
Good
Grateful
Confused
Sad
Ashamed
Lonely
Frustrated
Angry
Hurt
Jealous
Exhausted
Overwhelmed
Tired
Scared

I Spent most of today with

____
____
____
____
____

What I like the most today

____
____
____
____

What I like the least today

____
____
____

TODAY'S CHOICES

Physically	Mentally	Spiritually
☐ working	☐ reading	☐ meditating
☐ exercising	☐ doing a project	☐ praying
☐ shopping	☐ practicing	☐ with nature
☐ gardening	☐ organizing	☐ being challenged
☐ traveling	☐ thinking	☐ with family + friends
☐ playing	☐ planning	☐ relaxing

More thoughts...etc.....

SMTWTFS _________________ 20__ __ AM PM

☐ Sunny ☐ partly cloudy ☐ cloudy ☐ rain ☐ Snow

-10 zero 10's 20's 30's 40's 50's 60's 70's 80's 90's 100's
☐   ☐   ☐   ☐   ☐   ☐   ☐   ☐   ☐   ☐   ☐   ☐

I FEEL
Happy
Confident
Excited
Enthusiastic
Powerful
Fantastic
Lucky
Hopeful
Content
Focused
Good
Grateful
Confused
Sad
Ashamed
Lonely
Frustrated
Angry
Hurt
Jealous
Exhausted
Overwhelmed
Tired
Scared

I Spent most of today with

____

____

____

____

____

What I like the most today

____

____

____

____

What I like the least today

____

____

____

____

TODAY'S CHOICES

Physically	Mentally	Spiritually
☐ working	☐ reading	☐ meditating
☐ exercising	☐ doing a project	☐ praying
☐ shopping	☐ practicing	☐ with nature
☐ gardening	☐ organizing	☐ being challenged
☐ traveling	☐ thinking	☐ with family + friends
☐ playing	☐ planning	☐ relaxing

More thoughts...etc.....

SMTWTFS _________________________ 20___ ___ AM / PM

☐ Sunny ☐ partly cloudy ☐ cloudy ☐ rain ☐ Snow

-10 zero 10's 20's 30's 40's 50's 60's 70's 80's 90's 100's
☐   ☐   ☐   ☐   ☐   ☐   ☐   ☐   ☐   ☐   ☐   ☐

I FEEL
Happy
Confident
Excited
Enthusiastic
Powerful
Fantastic
Lucky
Hopeful
Content
Focused
Good
Grateful
Confused
Sad
Ashamed
Lonely
Frustrated
Angry
Hurt
Jealous
Exhausted
Overwhelmed
Tired
Scared

I Spent most of today with

____
____
____
____
____

What I like the most today

____
____
____
____

What I like the least today

____
____
____

TODAY'S CHOICES

Physically	Mentally	Spiritually
☐ working	☐ reading	☐ meditating
☐ exercising	☐ doing a project	☐ praying
☐ shopping	☐ practicing	☐ with nature
☐ gardening	☐ organizing	☐ being challenged
☐ traveling	☐ thinking	☐ with family + friends
☐ playing	☐ planning	☐ relaxing

More thoughts...etc.....

SMTWTFS _________________ 20___ ___

AM
PM

☐ Sunny ☐ partly cloudy ☐ cloudy ☐ rain ☐ Snow

-10 zero 10's 20's 30's 40's 50's 60's 70's 80's 90's 100's
☐   ☐   ☐   ☐   ☐   ☐   ☐   ☐   ☐   ☐   ☐   ☐

I FEEL
Happy
Confident
Excited
Enthusiastic
Powerful
Fantastic
Lucky
Hopeful
Content
Focused
Good
Grateful
Confused
Sad
Ashamed
Lonely
Frustrated
Angry
Hurt
Jealous
Exhausted
Overwhelmed
Tired
Scared

I Spent most of today with

____
____
____
____
____

What I like the most today

____
____
____
____

What I like the least today

____
____
____

TODAY'S CHOICES

Physically	Mentally	Spiritually
☐ working	☐ reading	☐ meditating
☐ exercising	☐ doing a project	☐ praying
☐ shopping	☐ practicing	☐ with nature
☐ gardening	☐ organizing	☐ being challenged
☐ traveling	☐ thinking	☐ with family + friends
☐ playing	☐ planning	☐ relaxing

More thoughts...etc.....

SMTWTFS _________________ 20___ ___   AM / PM

☐ Sunny   ☐ partly cloudy   ☐ cloudy   ☐ rain   ☐ Snow

-10 zero 10's 20's 30's 40's 50's 60's 70's 80's 90's 100's
☐   ☐   ☐   ☐   ☐   ☐   ☐   ☐   ☐   ☐   ☐   ☐

I FEEL
- Happy
- Confident
- Excited
- Enthusiastic
- Powerful
- Fantastic
- Lucky
- Hopeful
- Content
- Focused
- Good
- Grateful
- Confused
- Sad
- Ashamed
- Lonely
- Frustrated
- Angry
- Hurt
- Jealous
- Exhausted
- Overwhelmed
- Tired
- Scared

I Spent most of today with

____
____
____
____
____

What I like the most today

____
____
____
____

What I like the least today

____
____
____

TODAY'S CHOICES

Physically	Mentally	Spiritually
☐ working	☐ reading	☐ meditating
☐ exercising	☐ doing a project	☐ praying
☐ shopping	☐ practicing	☐ with nature
☐ gardening	☐ organizing	☐ being challenged
☐ traveling	☐ thinking	☐ with family + friends
☐ playing	☐ planning	☐ relaxing

More thoughts...etc.....

SMTWTFS _____________ 20__ __ AM / PM

☐ Sunny ☐ partly cloudy ☐ cloudy ☐ rain ☐ Snow

-10 zero 10's 20's 30's 40's 50's 60's 70's 80's 90's 100's
☐ ☐ ☐ ☐ ☐ ☐ ☐ ☐ ☐ ☐ ☐ ☐

I FEEL

- Happy
- Confident
- Excited
- Enthusiastic
- Powerful
- Fantastic
- Lucky
- Hopeful
- Content
- Focused
- Good
- Grateful
- Confused
- Sad
- Ashamed
- Lonely
- Frustrated
- Angry
- Hurt
- Jealous
- Exhausted
- Overwhelmed
- Tired
- Scared

I Spent most of today with

____

____

____

____

____

What I like the most today

____

____

____

____

What I like the least today

____

____

____

____

TODAY'S CHOICES

Physically	Mentally	Spiritually
☐ working	☐ reading	☐ meditating
☐ exercising	☐ doing a project	☐ praying
☐ shopping	☐ practicing	☐ with nature
☐ gardening	☐ organizing	☐ being challenged
☐ traveling	☐ thinking	☐ with family + friends
☐ playing	☐ planning	☐ relaxing

More thoughts...etc.....

SMTWTFS _________________ 20___ ___ AM / PM

☐ Sunny ☐ partly cloudy ☐ cloudy ☐ rain ☐ Snow

-10 zero 10's 20's 30's 40's 50's 60's 70's 80's 90's 100's
☐   ☐   ☐   ☐   ☐   ☐   ☐   ☐   ☐   ☐   ☐   ☐

I FEEL
- Happy
- Confident
- Excited
- Enthusiastic
- Powerful
- Fantastic
- Lucky
- Hopeful
- Content
- Focused
- Good
- Grateful
- Confused
- Sad
- Ashamed
- Lonely
- Frustrated
- Angry
- Hurt
- Jealous
- Exhausted
- Overwhelmed
- Tired
- Scared

I Spent most of today with

____
____
____
____
____

What I like the most today

____
____
____
____

What I like the least today

____
____
____

TODAY'S CHOICES

Physically	Mentally	Spiritually
☐ working	☐ reading	☐ meditating
☐ exercising	☐ doing a project	☐ praying
☐ shopping	☐ practicing	☐ with nature
☐ gardening	☐ organizing	☐ being challenged
☐ traveling	☐ thinking	☐ with family + friends
☐ playing	☐ planning	☐ relaxing

More thoughts...etc.....

Jiffy Journal

NOTES